Radical Self Love

Radical Self Love

An Ayurvedic Perspective on Health

Sandra Hayes
www.sandrahayes.eu

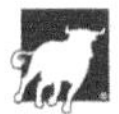

Troubador Publishing Ltd
Unit E2 Airfield Business Park
Harrison Road, Market Harborough
Leicestershire LE16 7UL
Tel: 0116 279 2299
Email: books@troubador.co.uk
Web: www.troubador.co.uk/matador

ISBN 978 1805141 310

British Library Cataloguing in Publication Data.
A catalogue record for this book is available from the British Library.

Typeset in 11pt Minion Pro by Troubador Publishing Ltd, Leicester, UK

Matador is an imprint of Troubador Publishing Ltd

With this book I hope to provide you with some inspiration and information that will help and empower you on your journey to better health and well-being.

It is, however, not my intention for you to take any of the given advice as a substitute for seeking medical attention or for taking prescribed medication. Please always seek the advice of your healthcare professional before making any changes to your prescribed medication or healthcare routine.

Contents

**SAMADOSHA SAMAGNISCHA
SAMADHATU MALAKRIYA
PRASANNA ATMENINDRIYA MANAHA
SWASTHYA ITYABHIDHYATE**

One whose Doshas, Agni and Dhatus are in balance, who properly eliminates all waste products, and whose true, authentic self, senses and mind are in a harmonious and pleasant state, is a truly healthy person.

(Ayurvedic definition of health, Sushrut Samhita, Chapter 15, Shloka 10)

Acknowledgements

I've written this book firstly for my own clients and students, and because I believe that in times like these it is more important than ever to take responsibility for our health. There is so much we can all do to prevent disease and live a happier, more balanced life in harmony with nature. It is, of course, not meant as medical advice or as a substitute for seeing a healthcare professional, if you are suffering from any health issues or symptoms.

It is purely meant as a supportive measure so that you can feel more empowered to listen to your own "gut" and begin to trust and love your body more.

I would like to thank my own teachers for empowering me to deepen my relationship with my own body and enable me to help others:

- Doug Hyde of Satmya Killaloe (www.satmya.ie)
- Dr Deepika Rodrigo and Dr Wathsala Wijesinghe of Ayurveda Institute UK (www.ayurvedainstitute. co.uk)
- Also, my own Ayurvedic practitioner, Dr Rajvinder

Kaur, who kindly wrote the foreword to this eBook and whose support I greatly value.

Dr Rajvinder Kaur BAMS attained her bachelor's degree in Ayurvedic Medicine and Surgery from Shri Krishna Government Ayurvedic College in the state of Haryana in India. This is a six-year degree course covering all aspects of Ayurvedic medicine. She has been working as an Ayurvedic practitioner in Ireland since 2007. For details check: www.ayurveda.ie.

Foreword

Rajvinder Kaur

Ayurveda's definition of "knowledge of life" offers us a beautiful insight into our health.

For good health, we need a strong digestive system and proper functioning of all parts of the body.

Ayurveda is a time-tested, evidence-based health system. It originated in India and is fully recognised by the World Health Organization (WHO). It is practised all over India and in many other countries and is rapidly establishing its place in the West.

Ayurveda is a prevention-based model, giving very successful results with chronic health conditions. It is a very gentle approach that is unique to everyone's individual constitution. Ayurveda looks at healing the whole person rather than fixing the symptoms. It teaches you how to nourish your mind and body by understanding your inner nature and connection with the power of nature around you. In this age and time, we are bombarded with many choices. Ayurveda focuses on diet, lifestyle and herbal preparations, as well as different healing therapies and yoga recommendations as per the health requirements of the person.

Sandra is a beautiful friend and a lovely person. She has put the knowledge of Ayurveda together in such a simplified way that makes it easy to understand. She has shared her own healing journey and experiences from an Ayurvedic point of view, which makes it inspiring for others.

Ayurveda says that health is not only a lack of physical symptoms, but also the balance of the physical, mental, emotional, environmental, and spiritual well-being of a person. It helps to see beyond the obstructions of life and to focus on self-love, self-care and the importance of unconditional love to reach your own maximum potential and allow the four main achievements (Dharma, Artha, Kama, Moksha) and purposes of human life to be fulfilled.

Health is the biggest wealth one can have. If we understand the principals of Ayurveda, it's very easy to incorporate them into our life.

First, we understand the make-up of our body in terms of Vata, Pitta and Kapha. Then we understand how nature operates within us and outside of the body in the form of circadian rhythms. By understanding this, we understand food better, as we are what we eat. If we provide Prana (vital energy) to our body as per our body type, we keep many diseases at bay, and if there is some imbalance, by following the basic principle, it becomes easy to bounce back.

By following simple rituals like self-massage, we keep our mind and body in harmony. Simple detox rituals at the change of seasons add vitality and rejuvenate our physiology. Daily routine and seasonal routine are a wonderful way of living. Ayurveda teaches us how to be in tune with nature and how to enjoy life with more awareness by connecting with our surroundings.

Many of my own patients find the connection between seasonal changes and the changes in their own body fascinating. It makes perfect sense that what is happening externally is reflected internally, and that understanding these environmental changes help them to operate more effectively in life.

Ayurveda puts you in charge of your own health and helps you lead a life full of health and happiness. You can achieve this by touching on the source of healing that lies within you and learn how to connect to it to be blissful all the time. As the Bhagavad Gita says:

"On this journey of life the body is the chariot, the mind is the driving instrument and intelligence is the driver operating through the five senses and you are the passenger."

Through the knowledge of Ayurveda, our intelligence learns how to skilfully drive the chariot and keep everything in harmony.

Through reading this book, you will gain much knowledge and have enough tools to stay healthy.

If you are working on some specific health issue, you can consult a well-trained Ayurveda practitioner.

Vaidya Rajvinder Kaur (B.A.M.S.)

Introduction

In May 1992, I went for a spin across Berlin on the back of my friend's motorbike. It was dark by the time we made our way home. Near a crossroad in the middle of the city, two kids suddenly came out of nowhere and ran across the road, forcing my friend to quickly turn his bike away.

We full-on hit a lamp post and I was catapulted 40 metres across the street – so I was told later. I sustained various life-threatening injuries, including an impalement through my perineum and abdomen and fractures to my pelvis. My friend died that night in the hospital.

I received surgery immediately to address my blood loss and spent two weeks on high doses of morphine in the emergency ward. Then I was moved into a general ward for the remainder of that summer.

Groups of students observed my body, and someone took pictures of my injuries for the medical books.

I was fitted with a colostomy bag and was told I'd have to live with it for the rest of my life.

Some of my teeth were gone too but I remember grinning through clouds of morphine at my friends, feeling oddly alive.

My friends had come to visit and pushed my bed into the hospital garden almost daily. They brought along instruments, and we sat outside under the weeping willows. I sang many toothless songs, accompanied by guitars and a saxophone. They dyed my hair with henna and brought me news from the outside world. I remember it as a good time.

By the end of the summer, I slowly started to walk again. Being young and restless, as soon as I felt the freedom of movement in my body, I left the hospital against the doctor's advice. Following the invitation of a friend, I left my crutches behind, and went travelling through Europe for a few weeks.

My spine and sacrum had been badly damaged but ,supported by my friends, I limped around the south of France, drank wine by the riversides, and learned to juggle at a circus festival in Spain.

Six months later, my colostomy bag was removed.

The doctors took pictures of me again, this time because I had healed so much better than anyone could have predicted.

Soon after, I went to study physical theatre and took tap dance, flamenco and belly dance classes.

Now, except for some scars and a stiffness in my left hip and knee, I have no lasting effects from the accident.

My body healed itself completely.

Why? Because that's what it was designed to do.

This experience was pivotal for me. It taught me a healthy respect for my life, and from this time onwards, I began to see my body – and the human body in general – with different eyes.

I recognised that it is not merely a machine, or some tool that moves us through life, which needs fixing every now and then, but that it is, in fact, a living organism, an expression of our deepest consciousness, a higher intelligence whose sole goal it is to keep us in a state of health so we can fulfill our higher purpose.

I learned that I needed to love my body in the same way I love my children – unconditionally.

The body is a self-healing organism.

It is incredibly capable of repairing the damage it experiences daily. Whether it is an accidental injury or trauma, or some other damage we inflict on it ourselves through our diet and lifestyle, the body will do anything in its power to return to a state of health and balance. We only have to let it.

All we must do is stop damaging it or at least slow down the rate of the damage enough for the healing mechanisms to be able to catch up.

If we just listened a little more to our body, if we learned how to read the subtle messages it is constantly giving us, treat it like the good friend it really is, we would be able to live a more deeply fulfilling life with a lot less suffering.

So, in this this book, I will try to give you the basic tools you need in order to learn to listen and understand the messages of your body again.

I will explain to you why looking after our digestion is the key to our health and how all of us can learn how to prevent and even reverse many disorders and diseases by simply changing our diet.

The human body is a perfect, intelligent, divine organism and it works tirelessly to keep us healthy, balanced and alive, so that we can live a happy and fulfilled life.

Once we understand this, we can begin to work with it, rather than against it. We can begin to love our bodies again.

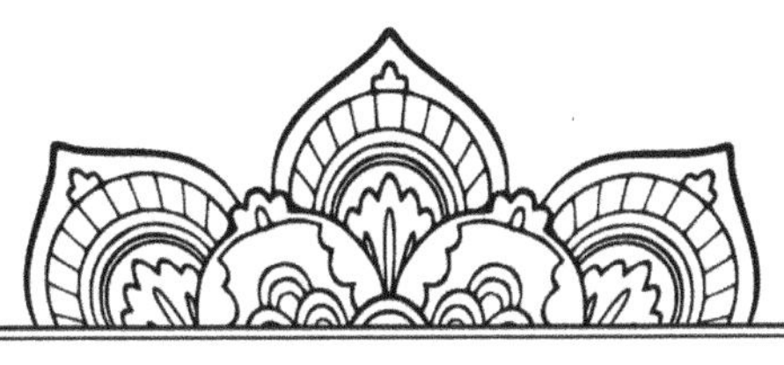

Part 1

About Ayurveda

What Is Ayurveda?

In Sanskrit, Ayu means life and Veda means knowledge. Ayurveda is the knowledge of life. But it is more than just biology. It is the wisdom of living – an age-old instruction manual that tells us exactly how we can live a joyful, vibrant, long and disease-free life.

It is a time-tested medical and healthcare system based on the ancient knowledge of the Vedas, whose vast and varied wisdom is as valid and effective today as it has been for over 5000 years. It gives us directions on how to prevent disease, improve our vitality, immunity and well-being, and relieve, and even reverse, many chronic illnesses and disorders.

It is a science that doesn't use high-powered microscopes, computers, or chemical solutions, and yet it is exceptionally accurate.

Its only measuring tools are our senses.

With our immediate perception of taste, sight, sound, touch, and smell, and through our own awareness and intuition, we can develop a true relationship with our biology, based on direct experience.

And all of us can learn it.

Ayurveda provides us with an ancient, yet new perspective for understanding a complex world in a holistic and easy way that empowers us to take responsibility for our own health and well-being.

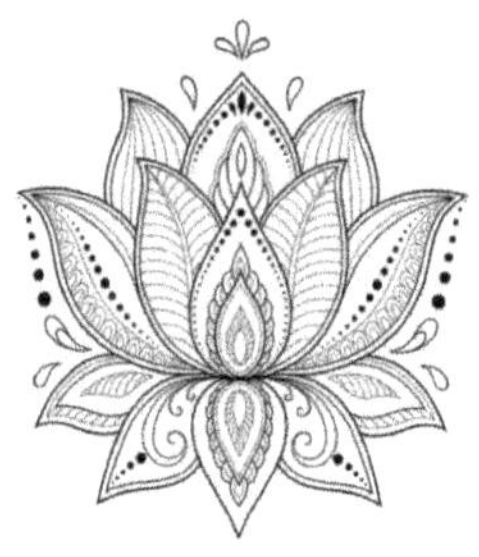

Samkhya –
A Philosophy of Love

Ayurveda is based on the principles of Samkhya. This is a branch of Vedic philosophy that describes the evolution of all that exists from pure consciousness to its manifested forms – pure energy, atoms, molecules and solid matter.

In contrast to our Western orthodox science, which until now believed that matter (the brain), generates consciousness, Ayurveda sees consciousness as the origin of everything that exists.

However, consciousness itself can only exist if it has something to be conscious of. This is the principle of duality that is reflected everywhere in nature: male and female, consciousness and body, intelligence and intuition are two sides of one reality and belong inseparably together. This duality is reflected in everything that exists, from the attraction of positive and negative particles, to the attraction between the male and female sex (or the male and female essence within us). This attraction is the basis of all life.

In Samkhya philosophy, this fundamental principle of duality is described as the divine masculine and feminine forces – the masculine represents consciousness (Purusha) and the feminine represents matter and energy (Prakrit). Prakriti is the matrix of the cosmos, the atomic particles that underlie everything that exists, and Purusha is the intelligence that moves them. Only when the two come together does life and individual consciousness arise.

This is beautifully described in the Vedic mythologies with their rich archetypal symbolism: Shiva and Shakti, the divine lovers, in their many forms and expressions; Brahma, the god of origination, who is orbited by his own feminine energy, which then manifests in all forms of nature; and Vishnu, the god of life and consciousness, who first falls asleep on a coiled serpent in the ocean of potentiality, before joining with the goddess Lakshmi to maintain the balance of nature.

These three divine pairs are allegories that stand for the three most fundamental of all qualities.

The Gunas – Primal Qualities of Nature

At the beginning of the 20th century, Einstein discovered and published the theory of relativity. This theory implies that energy is related to mass and the speed of light.

These three forces – energy, mass and light – are the fundamental forces of life. Prakriti (nature) is made up of these three constituents and we can see their properties and qualities within us and all around us, on every level of existence:

Rajas – the dynamic, fiery quality of energy, power and motivation can be observed in the growth of a plant or the striving of animals or humans to survive, reproduce and develop. It is the energy of spring, growth, wanting, learning and warmth. Movement generates this energy and since all life is constantly in motion, this is the energy that predominates our lives.

Tamas – the quality of mass, of inertia, is observable in the decay of plants and their return to the soil. It is also found in our own sleeping, dormant minds. It is the energy of autumn and winter, of earth and deep, dense soil, of stability and rest but also of strength and heaviness.

Sattva – the quality of light and expansion, enlightenment and lightness, as seen in the flowering of the plant, which gives off its fragrance and beauty, or in the fruit when it is perfectly ripe and sweet. It is also found in our own expanding consciousness, in our creativity, in the luminosity of our spirit that shines like the moon in the darkness.

The Dance of Desire

These qualities exist in everything, even in the smallest particles of matter, but they are not always active. In their purely potential, inactive state, they are in perfect equilibrium. In this state, before life begins, there is nothing needed, so there is no reason for activity. But as soon as this equilibrium is disturbed by a desire, a craving or a need for something, they come into motion and begin the rhythmic dance of life.

This desire is awakened, when the masculine principle of awareness merges with the feminine energy. When consciousness merges with matter, it becomes aware of itself.

In almost all cultures of the world, there are creation myths that describe this evolution in richt, symbolic images. Also the story of Adam and Eve contains this principle: Adam (Purusha) and Eve (Prakriti) are influenced by duality (the serpent) and become self-aware. Only then does individual consciousness arise and with it, the ego.

The gunas begin their dance of life:

*   When one is reduced, the other rises; when one becomes dominant, the other retreats.
*   We feel this effect ourselves in every moment: when we get hot, our body cools down by sweating; when we have overworked ourselves, we get tired, etc.
*   Every single one of our cells is thus constantly working to keep itself in balance.
*   Whenever there is a deficit, there is a desire to compensate for it. This is the basic principle of all evolution.

The marine animals, for example, one day experienced a deficit of food due to a natural disaster. The resulting desire caused them to move closer and closer to shallower areas, in search of nourishment. There, through the constant pressure of their fins against the ground, their muscles grew until at some point they were strong enough to move forward on land. Here, they strengthened even more, the muscles lengthening the bone, until the fins – over a long period of time – became legs.

The body always adapts to the inner deeds and the outer form always follows an inner desire.

From this perspective, life is really a constant dance of

causality – of action and reaction – with the aim of achieving a state of equilibrium. It is a dance of desire, caused by the need to create harmony.

Mahat – The Cosmic Intelligence

Samkhya philosophy describes the innate cosmic intelligence that exists in the molecular matrix and underlies nature throughout the universe – the force that moves us towards this state of equilibrium. Just as our heart knows how to beat, our cells know how to produce energy, and our skin, once injured, knows how to heal itself. The earth knows how to orbit the sun electrons know how to orbit the atomic nucleus. The force that keeps this cosmic dance in motion is controlled only by the need for harmony and love – by opposites attracting each other.

Only this need for unification of dualities and for a state of equilibrium of the gunas keeps our biological functions going.

The attraction of the polar opposites – consciousness and nature, Purusha and Prakriti, Shiva and Shakti, male and female, positive and negative energies – forms the primal drive of all of life.

And is this attraction, this longing of two opposing intelligent forces to merge and become one, nothing other than love?

I believe that love is the fundamental force that sets us and the entire universe in motion.

This cosmic force of love also lives in our bodies. Every single cell works tirelessly to fulfil its purpose, and this purpose is never limited to serving only itself. There is no ego in our body, only love and the intelligent power of nature. A cosmic intelligence that works for the good of the whole.

Our body never lies to us – it only ever tells us the truth about who we really are, about where we should go and about what we really need. And it has its very own language with which it communicates. If only we could understand it...

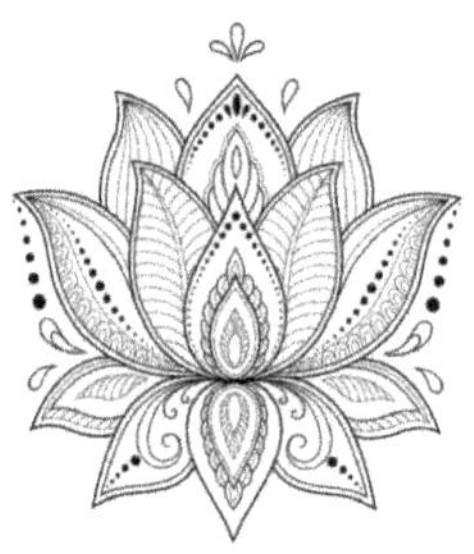

Ayurveda and Modern Medicine

Modern medicine has given us so much.

We have technologies that allow us to see the microscopic organisms inside our bodies, observe cells, and detect minuscule molecules. We have sophisticated methods of surgery, powerful medications that can suppress almost any painful or life-threatening symptom, and vaccines that have eradicated many diseases.

There is no doubt that our modern methods are working but, unfortunately, they come at a high price.

Side effects of medications are common and are even the third leading cause of death in the US according to a 2018 study.

And while many, mostly infectious, diseases are now history, thanks to modern knowledge, many others are on the rise, like allergies, auto-immune diseases, cancer, heart disease, and diabetes.

Our life expectancy has increased and our risk of injury and infection has decreased but still we are no closer to achieving optimal health than we were at any other time. In fact, in many cases, it seems to be getting worse each year.

It looks like, while we are living longer, we are also getting significantly sicker.

According to the WHO, chronic disease in 2001 accounted for 60% of deaths worldwide. That's a staggering number, especially since many chronic diseases are a result of lifestyle and diet and could therefore be preventable.

But with the growth of possibilities in medicine also comes more responsibility for our doctors to know their way around all the different medications.

As more and more new medications are being approved, education about their use and side effects takes up more and more time of the five to six years a medical student spends at university, leaving less and less time for diet and nutrition, and the actual prevention of these diseases.

Simply, the roles of our doctors have changed.

If we need to address acute, life-restricting, or even life-threatening issues, a surgeon or GP will be able to prescribe effective drugs to counteract your symptoms so you can regain some quality of life.

But it is simply no longer his or her role to make sure that you are eating well, exercising, and living a generally healthy life to support your body's self-healing mechanisms and to prevent those issues from arising in the first place.

This responsibility is all yours.

But how can we take this responsibility if we don't know much about nutrition either? If most of the information about our food comes from advertisements and from biased studies sponsored by the food industry, how can we be expected to find our way through the thousands of conflicting messages we are hearing, from superfoods to super diets, supplements, and ads for chocolate bars?

Many scientific studies nowadays are funded by companies with a vested interest in their outcome. It is not difficult to manipulate such studies but it is hard for a layperson to make real sense of the information that is available for us.

And we can't all become nutrition experts, can we?

And besides, what's said to be good for us seems to be changing all the time. When I was a child growing up, milk, meat and bread were the most precious foods anyone could. Now they seem to be the most condemned, replaced by kale smoothies and chia seeds.

What is there to do if we want to regain control over our health?

We can't keep handing over all responsibilities to our healthcare systems, blame the advertisements and false studies, and expect our doctors to fix the problems we are unwittingly inflicting on ourselves.

If only we had some kind of guidance on how to understand the messages of our bodies better so we can recognise what it really needs…

Enter Ayurveda!

Ayurveda is a system that teaches us exactly that – how to understand what our body really needs and how we can recognise early stages of imbalances easily so that we can do something about it.

And it doesn't have to be complicated at all.

A Holistic Science

While modern science takes the reductionistic approach of analysing and separating, dividing the whole into its smallest parts in order to understand them, Ayurveda takes the approach of synthesis, of putting the parts back together to recognise a whole, living organism that functions in constant communication with its surroundings.

I'm not pitching one against the other here. To be able to see the tiniest detail of a living organism and observe even the smallest particle is extremely valuable and has led us to so many interesting and life-altering discoveries but to look at a small detail for too long sometimes makes us forget the bigger picture.

It's like trying to get to know a bird by cutting it into pieces vs studying its behaviour.

Or, as the German saying goes, we lose sight of the woods because of all the trees.

It's fine to be proud of and grateful for our scientific discoveries – after all, they have saved so many lives that would have otherwise been lost to accidents and diseases – but let's not forget that many, if not most, of these diseases could have been prevented in the first place. And saving a life doesn't necessarily mean increasing the quality of that life, or its happiness, energy and joy.

I believe that modern science and the ancient methods of Ayurveda can work wonderfully together.

It is like merging the dual forces of the divine masculine and feminine, analysis and synthesis, quantity and quality, emergency medicine and disease prevention.

The linear, academic approach of the masculine, who experiences the world through the mind, and the non-linear feminine, who experiences the world through the senses, experience and intuition. One alone is not enough to truly understand life. We need both, together.

If I have a toothache, I will not hesitate to take a painkiller, and I will be grateful for it. But if I get frequent tooth infections, taking painkillers each time will not change the cause of the problem. It may even put an extra strain on my liver and affect its healthy functioning in the long run.

If we get frequent headaches, we can take a painkiller each time until we feel better. But if we never ask ourselves why we get the headaches in the first place, they may just keep coming back and, eventually, they will turn into something worse.

Of course, suppressing symptoms isn't a bad thing in itself – it can be life-saving at times – but ignoring the causes of a disease is eventually going to catch up with us.

Most of us are used to ignoring the body's subtle messages.

Only when the discomfort we are in becomes greater than the fear of having to make a change will many of us be ready to take responsibility.

In Western medicine, the first stage of disease is the display of symptoms.

In Ayurveda, the display of symptoms is the fourth stage.

Long before the first symptoms manifest, the body gives us subtle signs of imbalance. Ayurveda teaches us how to read those signs and trace back the pathways of the disease to its origins, so we can make appropriate changes in our lives. And when we do, the body will regain balance all by itself, because that is what it is designed to do.

We can all learn to read these signs. We can all create a better, deeper relationship with our body, like a best friend who is there to guide us through our lives.

It is simply a matter of learning to look through a new

lens, to gain a fresh perspective on what our body actually is: a living organism, full of life, intelligence, and love.

"There is no combination of medications that can bring harmony to over 280,000 different protein structures and millions of protein and hormone pathways that orchestrate human health."
Zach Bush MD

"The body heals itself. It can do so because it has a healing system."
Andrew Weil M.D.

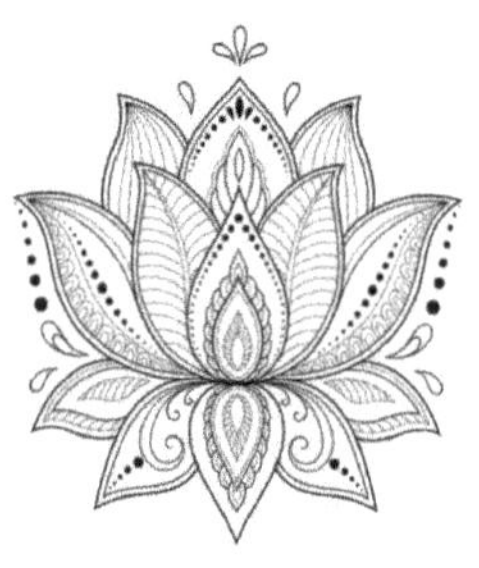

The Five Elements

Ayurveda recognises the body not as a fixed object, nor a machine, but as a living organism that is in constant communication with its surroundings. Its internal structure is continually moving, fluctuating, and changing with each internal or external influence. It is literally like a dance that happens inside every organ and every cell of our body, even on a molecular level.

If the outside temperature is hot, the body cools down by moistening the skin with sweat from its sweat glands.

If the internal hydration levels go down, our nervous system communicates thirst, and we go and get ourselves a glass of water.

And once we drink the water, it filters through our kidneys and flushes out any accumulated toxins on its way out through the bladder.

As much as we may take our body's functions for granted, we have to admit that it is quite a miraculous, incredibly intelligent organism. And it never stops. It never stays still, not even in our sleep.

Life is continuous movement. There is no such thing as

stillness, but stillness is the ultimate aim of all movement. This brings us back to the balance of the Gunas – the inherent, basic qualities of all matter – and the merging of the dual opposites – the negative and positive charge, or the masculine and feminine.

To find the perfect point of equilibrium is the constant aim of our body.

And, in its continuous fluctuation, our body is never quite the same. Just like a flowing river, it constantly changes and its needs are different at any given time.

Also, nobody is the same as the next.

These differences mean that each of us will respond slightly – but significantly – differently to outside influences.

You may have noticed these kinds of differences between you and the people around you. Maybe you get cold easily and like to turn up the heat at the beginning of September while your husband sits near the open window in his T-shirt, dabbing beads of sweat off his face. You may have noticed how, although you have no diagnosed gluten intolerance, you might feel bloated from eating bread while your son can eat whole loaves of it without any adverse reaction.

Or maybe you put on weight easily even though you eat less than your skinny friend who never even exercises.

Of course, we are all different.

Each of us is a divine expression of a mere aspect of the infinite whole.

And it's in our subtle differences, that we can find the clues to understanding our physiological and psychological makeup, and to finding our way towards optimal health and vitality, and a more joyful experience of life.

How Does It Work?

A fixed object can be named but how do you describe something that is constantly changing?

It is simple.

We don't use fixed nouns, but adjectives instead.

If I tried to describe my friend to you, I wouldn't use nouns. If I just told you her name, it wouldn't mean a thing to you. If I told you that she has hair and hands and feet, a liver and a heart, you probably wouldn't find her very interesting and you certainly wouldn't feel like you could understand her personality and nature. But if I told you that her hair is beautiful, long and brown, that her laugh sounds like trickling water, that she has a sharp mind and an inquisitive nature and is fiercely passionate about her goals in life, you probably have a much better picture of her already, and maybe you feel that she somehow becomes interesting to you.

It's the adjectives that describe her personality, her inner qualities, and the nature of her true self.

It's the same with the human body. Our bodies too have different kinds of personalities. They are expressions of our souls. They , too, need adjectives to describe their qualities in a way we truly can grasp.

There are, of course, a large number of adjectives but, to simplify it, Ayurveda uses 20 of them to describe our bodily substances:

COLD – HOT

SLOW – SHARP

OILY – DRY

CLEAR – ADHESIVE

SUBTLE – GROSS

STATIC – MOBILE

HEAVY – LIGHT

DENSE – LIQUID

SMOOTH – ROUGH

SOFT – HARD

The above-mentioned qualities can be symbolically summarised into five elements:

EARTH
Cold, dull, coarse, static, dense, hard

WATER
Cold, clear, mobile, fluid, smooth, soft, heavy

FIRE
Hot, cutting, mobile, subtle, light

AIR
Cold, dry, mobile, subtle, rough

ETHER
Dry, clear, subtle, light, clear

Pancha Mahabhuta

(Pancha = Five, Maha = Great, Bhuta = Essence)

A large part of Eastern philosophy and medicine is based on the idea that every kind of matter can be reduced to these five basic essences (Pancha = five, Mahabhuta = basic essences). All molecules can therefore be divided into these elementary groupings. This means that everything in nature has certain properties that correspond in different variations to those of earth, water, fire, air and/or ether.

The properties of the molecules of the element earth are generally large, heavy, slow, immobile, hard or coarse and form heavy, dense mass.

The properties of molecules of the element water are essentially fluid, smooth, cold, heavy and mobile, and form the fluids of nature as well as in our bodies.

Molecules of the element fire are heat-producing, decomposing (cutting), transforming, consuming, mobile and light and are found in acids and enzymes, while the molecules of air correspond to light, gaseous molecules and communicative frequencies, like the firing of synopsis.

All these elements are contained in the ether, which is the space in which they move. This space is vast, subtle, clear and light, and it expands according to its content.

In this way we can describe all manifested life on earth.

For example, if a person has a higher proportion of earth element in his or her body than others, then this means that this person very likely has denser cell tissue and more body mass than others, which may also lead to a certain heaviness and slowness of synapses and metabolism. This person would then likely also be outwardly slower, in speech, thought and action, but would probably possess good muscular strength and a stable nervous system. Someone with more etheric elements might have a lighter bone structure and more mobile joints due to the larger cavities. His cell structure could be much more permeable than that of other people. Nutrients and messages from the nervous system are thus transported more quickly, which means that these people can be extremely sensitive, not only to physical touch, but also to sounds, feelings and experiences.

Someone with more fire qualities, on the other hand, probably has a particularly strong metabolism because of the greater heat-producing, enzymatic activity. This person digests much more than others, both physically and mentally.

The heat in his body and the light receptors in his skin may cause him to be sensitive to light and hot temperatures. Perhaps these people suffer from inflammation or hyperacidity more often than others.

A person who has a lot of watery substances in her body will certainly appear more hydrated on the outside than others. She may have smoother skin, thick hair and beautiful, shining eyes. In addition, she very likely also produces a greater proportion of sexual fluids, tears and urine.

And a person with the characteristics of the air element may tend to have more movement in the body, such as transports in the nervous system, peristalsis, blood circulation, etc.. He or she may have a preference to move a lot or talk, or think a lot. He or she may grasp things quickly and forget them just as easily. He or she will probably feel the need for freedom more strongly than others. The consistency of hair and skin, as well as the sense of humour, will often be drier than others.

This way of categorising our differences allows us to understand and describe our innermost being in a much more vivid and life-affirming way.

When we use this kind of terminology, we discover that the five basic elements together describe three basic kinds of energies or substances in our bodies:

* Our body mass (tissues, bones, mucous membranes, water content), which is a combination of the properties of mostly water and some earth.
* The energy that our body produces and uses (metabolism, enzyme secretions, body temperature), which is a combination of the properties of mainly fire and some water.
* The movement by which all activities are carried out (circulation, nerve impulses, peristalsis, etc.), which is a combination of the properties of air and ether.

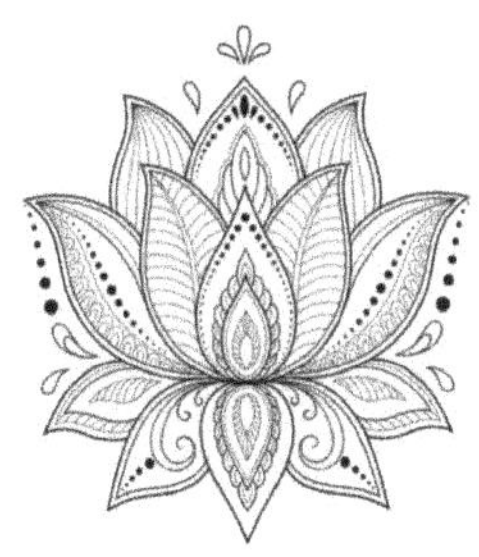

The Doshas

These three categories are used in Ayurveda to understand the human body.

The different amounts in which we all possess these three essential constituents determines our individual physiological constitution.

In Ayurveda, they are called the three doshas: Kapha, Pitta and Vata.

Dosha actually means "fault" or "that which causes disease". It is a clear indication of our strengths and weaknesses, both physically and mentally. We are all made up of the five elements, but in different compositions. The elements that predominate in us may produce our strengths, but they can also easily turn into weaknesses if they get out of balance.

Just as we take care of our own children, we must also respond to our Dosha: a child who loves to snuggle up to us, read or watch TV while eating chocolate needs to be encouraged to eat vegetables and be physically active sometimes. A child who always wants to run around outside needs to be gently encouraged to rest, and a child who is competitive and likes to get involved in hobbies or sports may need to be calmed down more often.

The different substances and qualities of our body-mind-organism can be explained very well with the concept of the doshas:

Vata

Vata is a combination of the elements of air and space, which form the light, dry, moving, subtle components of the body. This is expressed in bodily functions like the circulation of blood and nervous impulses (Vyana Vata), the peristalsis and microbial activity in the gut (Samana Vata), the intake of oxygen and life force through breath and nourishment (Prana Vata), the elimination of carbon dioxide through exhaling and the expression of our voice (Udana Vata), and the elimination of waste products through menstruation, urine and faeces (Apana Vata).

People who possess a lot of Vata qualities often have, just like the elements of air and space, a natural tendency to be lighter and thinner than others. Their body shape is often long-limbed and tall, or sometimes particularly small. The irregularity of Vata shows up in asymmetrical features, protruding joints, and unruly hair, while dryness produces fine, frizzy hair and dry skin. The movement aspect of air gives quick nervous impulses – they react much more sensitively than others to sensual input. They also often have an urge to move a lot, be it in the form of walking, running, or other types of physical movement, or in the form of travelling. They don't like sitting still and are drawn to new impressions frequently. Sometimes the moving aspect of this

Dosha shows up more in the mind, in the form of excessive thinking or speaking, or daydreaming and fantasising. Air and space can make them light, free and independent but also ungrounded and nervous. They are quick learners but tend to forget information just as quickly again. They are the rebels among us, thinking differently and outside the box. There are many artists, free thinkers and revolutionaries among them. And as much as we need rebels in our lives, without them there would be no change and life would stagnate. Too much Vata can easily cause trouble.

As Vata is the most unstable of the Doshas, it is easy to accumulate and get out of balance. When the natural flow of movement in the body is disturbed in any way, we can develop many problems – constipation, bloating, circulatory issues, nervous system disorders, and mental health issues. We can become anxious and nervous or suffer from nutritional deficiencies.

The Ayurvedic textbooks list 80 different types of diseases that are associated with Vata Dosha, 40 for Pitta, and 20 for Kapha. Once Vata is out of balance, unless we bring it back, it can disturb all other Doshas and invite more trouble than necessary.

Dehydration of our cell membranes – often caused by stress – will prevent nutrients to be properly absorbed and energy metabolism to be disturbed. This is the basis for many problems we might develop.

Thankfully, there are plenty of ways we can keep our Vata in check. One of the best methods to calm, nourish and soothe the nervous system, support circulation and counteract the drying qualities of Vata, is the routine of a daily oil massage, which I will describe later on.

Pitta

Pitta is the combination of fire and water, which, like hot oil or boiling water, stands for everything burning, hot, consuming, and transforming in our bodies. Mostly, this means stomach acid and enzymes in the stomach and duodenum (Pachaka Pitta), enzymes, bile and red blood cells in the liver (Ranjaka Pitta), the intelligence of our heart and brain (Sadhaka Pitta), which processes information, the light receptors in our eyes (Alochaka Pitta) and the colour and sun-sensitivity in our skin (Bhrajaka Pitta).

Because of the hot, transformative quality of fire, people with a Pitta constitution have a lot of metabolic heat in their bodies. They are the types of people who are often hungry and need their regular meals or they will get irritable and "hangry". If they are otherwise in good health, they can digest almost anything and tend to neither lose nor gain weight easily. The light of the fire influences their appearance too. Often they are quite fair in skin tone (compared to others of the same ethnicity) and have light or strongly coloured eyes and hair. They are quite sensitive to the sun. The balance between fire and water shows in a balanced appearance and a medium, usually well-formed body shape.

It also gives them a balance between strength and flexibility, which means that they are generally good at most forms of exercise and make good athletes. Their sense of achievement can, at times, make them quite competitive.

They digest not only food well, but also experiences and information too. Bright and intelligent with a well-developed discerning quality, they come across as extremely intelligent and confident.

Whatever they do, they seem to excel at it. This is because they fully immerse themselves in any task at hand. They are passionate about all sorts of aspects of their lives, from their work, their children, and their romantic partners to their spiritual beliefs and moral convictions.

Pitta-type people are natural-born leaders and teachers. Like fire, they shine brightly and radiate their knowledge, warmth, and passion out into the world.

But if Pitta rises too high, their passion can easily turn into anger, control issues or obsessions and they can become quite arrogant and competitive. They can be prone to digestive issues like acid reflux, ulcers, and diarrhoea.

Pitta needs to keep the delicate balance between its own elements of water and fire, as fire can easily turn into inflammation. When Pitta is out of balance for a long time, issues like rheumatoid arthritis, rashes, infections, migraines, and premature greying or balding might emerge.

Keeping Pitta cool with cooling foods and soothing activities is important particularly to those who already have a natural Pitta constitution with high amounts of fire.

One of the best ways, in my opinion, to keep Pitta in check is meditation. To sit and concentrate on our breath or some other object of our meditation uses the Pitta person's natural tendency to focus as a way to calm and cool the mind and body. There are many wonderful ways to learn techniques of meditation – all it takes is a few minutes of practice every day to feel the results.

Another way to ease the heating effect of Pitta is to focus on what gives you joy. It may sound like a cliche but especially for people with a Pitta aggravation, it can be very important to remember all the small joys in life to help them ease away from trying to be in control of things all the time. Having fun occasionally, going to a spa or concert or to watch a silly movie can be just as important as doing our daily work.

Kapha

Kapha is a combination of earth and water. Like fertile soil or mud, it is sticky and dense. As mucus membranes, it coats the linings of the stomach (Kledaka Kapha), lubricates and protects nerve endings in the brain (Tarpaka Kapha), lubricates and nourishes joints (Sleshaka Kapha), moistens food and activates taste buds and digestion (Bodhaka Kapha), and protects the lungs and heart (Avalambaka Kapha).

Earth and Water give people with a natural Kapha constitution a strong body with a well-lubricated skin and membranes. You can see it in their often broad, muscular, chubby, or curvy shape and their soft, smooth, and plump skin. They tend to have thick, lush hair and shiny eyes. Even their personalities are well lubricated – soft-spoken, with a pleasant, soothing voice and a calming, smooth mannerism, they seem attractive to others and are well-liked by many. They form attachments easily and make loyal friends and devoted partners or parents. They are often traditional and like to stick to things they know. The nourishing, adhesive qualities of water give them the urge to nurture.

Their nervous system membranes too are well formed and they can deal with a lot of pressure in life, so much that, given their kind and caring nature, they often are taken advantage of. But they are no pushover either.

A passage from *The Penelopiad* by Margaret Atwood, puts it perfectly into words:

"Water does not resist. Water flows. When you plunge your hand into it, all you feel is a caress. Water is not a solid wall, it will not stop you. But water always goes where it wants to go, and nothing, in the end, can stand against it. Water is patient. Dripping water wears away a stone. Remember that, my child. Remember you are half water. If you can't go through an obstacle, go around it. Water does."

Kapha people are the most patient of all constitutions. They are rarely in a rush and, in fact, they dislike being rushed. They take their sweet time with almost everything. At times, it makes them seem as if they are a little dull or unintelligent but, although it is true that they take in information more slowly, they actually retain it better than anyone. Like elephants, they never forget. They are emotional people and learn best when they feel emotionally connected, through stories for example, or personal experience.

Although they are extremely sensual beings and enjoy all pleasures of the senses, including food, they could easily go without food for a long time. Due to their slow metabolism, they do better on just one or two meals a day instead of the usual three. If they eat the same amount as their Pitta-type friends, they will easily put on unwanted weight.

Kapha imbalances can also show up as increased mucus production, which can result in coughs, colds, blocked sinuses, etc.

It sometimes shows up in the form of swollen joints or water retention in the legs, and other issues of accumulation in the body, like high cholesterol, high blood sugar, diabetes, weight gain or fibroids.

One of the most important things for Kapha people is to leave enough time between meals for digestion – as much time as needed until real hunger occurs again – as well as regular exercise. It's easy for a Kapha person to stay on the couch and watch TV; it can be hard for them to get going. But once they do, they have great stamina and can workout or walk for hours.

Of course, it's important to pick an exercise that is enjoyable and can actually be sustained, and for Kapha people this might mean connecting exercise with beauty. Salsa or belly dancing will probably suit them well or walking in nature. Yoga or weightlifting are also great choices as they utilise their natural strength and stamina.

Tri-Dosha

Each of us, of course, is an expression of all three Doshas – Vata, Pitta and Kapha. However, they are never equally balanced.

One or two of them always more or less dominate, and so are determining individual types of digestion, metabolism, physical appearance, function, and personality.

As you read through the descriptions, you may recognise yourself most clearly in one or two of these types, although our constitution can fluctuate and be influenced by many different factors.

For example, when we are children, we all have a higher amount of Kapha Dosha. Our water content is higher (about 75%) and our bodies are growing and gaining in mass every day. We are attached to our parents and full of love. When we get out of balance, it often is shown in an over-production of mucus – runny noses, chest infections, etc. And we love the taste of sweet things.

During adolescence, when hormonal activities light the fire of Pitta, we become more passionate and discerning. We become more focused on who we are or who we want to be; we are more analytical and often also more aggressive and assertive. Our taste preferences change and our imbalances are more due to an abundance of Pitta, such as inflammation, allergies, acne, etc.

During most of our adult life, we remain in this Pitta-dominated phase, governed by fertility and productivity. We work, study, and focus on our tasks in life. And then, when we get older, our fertility dries up and our productive endeavours slow down. Often we begin to have an urge to do something creative with our lives – write a book or take art classes or tell stories to our grandkids. At this time, the water content in our bodies is only at about 55% – we have entered the Vata phase of our lives. We become the elders, the wise ones, preparing for letting go of life. In the great process of digesting our life, this is the time of elimination. We give back what we don't need anymore, so that others can be nourished. We give our wisdom to the world.

So, through the influences of time, our constitution changes.

Also, the seasons, our climate, what we eat, the people around us, our experiences, and even the time of day all influence the fluctuations of our Dosha. At midday, for example, when the sun is high, our digestive fire is also high, which is why it is best to eat the biggest meal of the day for lunch.

Most of the time, we naturally react to these fluctuations.

In winter, when it is cold, we dress warmer and turn up the heat. When we are hungry, we eat; when we feel stressed or tired, we rest; and we avoid people or situations who aggravate us in some way.

But sometimes, be it because we aren't aware enough or because of outside pressures, we let things influence us for too long.

Sometimes, we remain in a bad relationship for too long, or in a job we don't like, or we keep eating the same kind of food we know causes us digestive issues. Perhaps we've moved to a colder climate from a warm and sunny place and find it difficult to adjust. And so, the aggravations grow, slowly and steadily, into imbalances of our body and mind.

The sooner we react to any aggravating circumstances, the easier it is to counteract imbalances and avoid more serious issues. The trick is to learn how to listen to the body's signs more carefully, recognising its messages before it is too late.

Prakruti
(Nature/Creation – Our Genetic Constitution)

Of course, we have certain genetic traits we've inherited from our parents that we simply can't change.

We may have inherited the genetic markers for diabetes or heart disease and, especially if we continue our family traditions of rich, heavy food, we may be likely to develop them.

But whether or not these traits will be activated during our lifetime depends on many other factors we can actually control.

Ayurveda recognises that Prakruti, our individual nature, is determined by our inherited genetics, by our karma, by the time and place of conception, the time and place of birth, and also by the emotional and physical state our parents were in during conception, pregnancy, and birth.

Karma, in Sanskrit, means "action" and refers to the causality of life. Every action gives rise to a reaction and is, at the same time, the consequence of a previous action. If I asked you to tell me exactly why you are sitting here, reading this book at this very moment, if I asked you to trace back your original impulse, the original cause of your current action, how far back would the sequence of events bring you? If you really traced back the actions all the way to the source, chances are that you are going to end up at your birth. And we could even go back further than that, asking what karma may have caused us to be born in this time and place.

Life is, in truth, a big web of actions and reactions not only of you but of all other beings around you.

There are countless influences that play an important role in our lives. And they have all led to us being exactly where we are right now, in this very moment, in all our physical, mental and emotional glory.

Some of us were conceived under rather unfortunate circumstances, for example by a mother who didn't actually want to have a child and harboured a secret resentment of our existence during her pregnancy. Even if she did her best to hide these feelings, they will have affected our developing subconscious mind. It is even likely that because of this our lives have been marked by the subliminal conviction of being unwanted, rejected or unworthy.

This subtle feeling – unpleasant as it may be – often

becomes the cornerstone of our own destiny: it is our life's mission to grow beyond these feelings, to free ourselves from these particular karmic patterns, that were probably carried for generations, or across previous lives. And in order to resolve these patterns, we have to become aware of them. So, our unconscious mind will present us with these emotions, triggered by different situations we will find ourselves in, again and again, repeatedly causing us to feel rejected and undesirable, until we have finally transcended them.

It is our dharma, our evolutionary task, our mission in this life on the path of spiritual growth to outgrow such constricting beliefs, to free ourselves from unconscious conditioning and to become aware of our true nature. Only then can we actually be healthy and happy.

However, it is not only the feelings of the parents, but also the environment and the special time and place of conception and birth that influence our prakruti. The particular constellation of the stars, the phase of the moon, the season, the age of our parents and even the time of day all form our subconscious mind and thus our developing physiology.

Let me give you an example of this.

My family on my mother's side has many Kapha characteristics. All my aunts, uncles and cousins have thick, dark, mostly curly hair and big brown eyes. They love to eat and take care of their families. Every time they get together, it's all about food. There is a lot of love expressed. However, my parents were teenagers when I was conceived; it was high summer and I was born around midday. All these Pitta qualities had an impact on my foetal development and eventually gave me my own Kapha-Pitta constitution – I am the only one in the family who freckles in summer.

Our prakruti creates the foundation for our health and sets the tone for how we communicate with our environment, digest our food and deal with life in general. It shows us our innate strengths and weaknesses.

If we want to live a truly harmonious life, we need to respect and appreciate our individual constitution.

Of course, I have inherited my family's Kapha tendencies. This is evident in my glucose metabolism, among other things. A DNA test has confirmed that I am prone to diabetes, but by eating a largely Kapha-balanced diet I can prevent this.

When I moved to Ireland in the 1990s, where it's cold and wet, my Kapha constitution became a bit imbalanced. For a while I got frequent respiratory infections and also gained weight until I finally learned about Ayurveda and found my balance by adopting a Kapha-reducing diet and lifestyle. Maintaining my weight and avoiding diabetes or other disorders is not difficult as long as I know my Dosha and what my body needs. When we respect ourselves as we are and treat ourselves well, we also have much more energy and feel good all around.

Emotionally, it is also important to respect ourselves as we naturally are.

A Vata child, for example, will never be able to sit still as long as a Kapha child and a Kapha child will never do his homework as efficiently as a Pitta child. It does us no good to complain that we can't eat as much as our best friend without gaining weight – if we want to feel good in our bodies, we simply have to respect our individual metabolism as it is.

Vikruti ("After Creation") – Our Imbalances

As mentioned before, we are in continuous communication and exchange of energy with our environment. Our mind-body organism is always trying to maintain its equilibrium by adapting to external influences.

Just like we dress warmer when the weather turns cold and we eat when we are hungry, the internal environment of our body also reacts to any influences (internal or external) by either increasing or decreasing certain qualities to maintain equilibrium – if it is cold outside, our internal body temperature rises; if we get too hot, sweat glands are activated, and so on.

But what would happen if we didn't dress warmly when it was cold? If we take a long walk on a cold winter's day in our T-shirts, we are very likely to get sick.

If, in an attempt to counteract the external cold (Vata), our internal heat (Pitta) is turned up so much that we end up with inflamed tissues, and our mucus production (Kapha) is increased to soothe the inflammation, we will begin to cough and sneeze, develop a fever and generally feel very unwell.

But what if it isn't as obvious as this example?

What happens if these Dosha aggravations happen slowly and subtly?

If, for example, you go for walks in the wind a lot. Maybe you like to eat a lot of cold foods, like salads, and dry snacks such as nuts and crackers. Maybe you run around and talk a lot all day or work irregular hours or night shifts and don't get to rest adequately, or you go out at night until the morning hours, drink alcohol and coffee, or spend a lot of time travelling or moving house.

All these influences will cause stress in your nervous system and gradually increase the Vata qualities in your body, especially if you already are of a predominantly Vata constitution.

You may not immediately get sick but, slowly, these Vata qualities will accumulate. You might notice a little more bloating, maybe some headaches. Your energy levels are a little low. Maybe you feel more nervous or anxious than you used to. Maybe you feel tired a lot. Or your sleep becomes light. And if nothing changes, if you keep running in the wind, staying up at night, eating cold, dry food, and juggling too many things at once, the accumulated Vata will spread through your body and settle anywhere where there is a weak spot.

The dryness might move into your joints, making them crack and feel stiff, and may eventually develop into arthritis. Perhaps it will affect your skin, causing dryness and flaky eczema, or it might develop into a migraine.

Also our cell membranes will, if they become dehydrated, not function properly and cause our nutrient assimilation and energy production to be impaired.

If we can recognise the signs long before a disease has manifested, we can treat it and restore it back to balance.

If we understand the difference between our actual constitution (Prakruti) and the state of our body that has been acquired through life's influencing factors (Vikruti), we can read the signs much more clearly and react accordingly.

Our Vikruti can change significantly over time. We may be a natural Kapha-type person but Vata or Pitta can dominate our physiology during certain phases of our life, depending on our age, diet, lifestyle and environment.

This basic concept is important to understand, as all diseases originate in one or more simple changes in the body's natural constitution.

And of course, as all of us are different to begin with, our tendencies to develop certain disorders vary too.

A person born with a lot of Kapha qualities (low metabolism, high mucus productivity, etc.), who lives in a cold, wet place and eats a lot of heavy, sweet, or fatty foods, all of which will further increase Kapha, will easily become overweight or develop issues like asthma or blocked sinuses, cholesterol or diabetes, while a person with a Vata or Pitta constitution might get away with the same kind of diet without developing any problems.

However, a Pitta-type person in a high-pressure job, eating a lot of spicy foods, will be much more likely to develop digestive problems like stomach ulcers, acid reflux, diarrhoea or inflammatory diseases, and burn out, while the Kapha person can easily deal with the same things. A sensitive Vata person will be much more easily traumatised by a threatening situation than a Kapha or a Pitta person.

Our bodies are always in communication with our environment, and they are continuously giving us messages about how they are coping.

And, as opposed to our minds, our bodies do not have an ego-based agenda. They do not lie. They always speak the truth.

All we have to do is pay attention.

Once we understand that, we are truly empowered to become the creators of our own lives.

Of course, there are still a lot of factors outside our immediate control, like genetics and environmental influences, so we cannot always avoid becoming sick. However, for the most part, we already know that cancer, chronic diseases and many other disorders are, to a large extent, preventable by diet and lifestyle.

By simply increasing our awareness and respect for our own body and natural constitution, we can experience big changes in our lives.

Changes that will lead to greater health and well-being, more energy and vibrancy, and a more fulfilled, happy life.

And it all begins with our digestion.

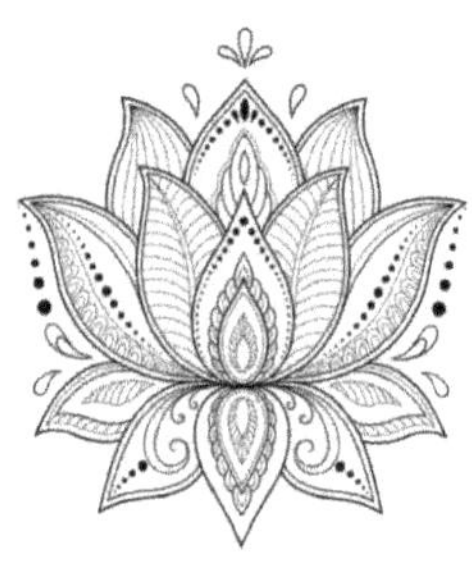

Part 2

Digestion & Immunity

Why Digestion Is the Base of Good Health

The body is a self-regulating, self-healing organism.

When we cut our skin, as long as we can keep it reasonably clean, it will heal itself. If we get infected by a virus, the immune system works tirelessly to overcome it and restore the body's health.

Our hearts beat all by themselves, our lungs breathe because of the automatic response of the diaphragm, and any toxins that may have entered the body are flushed out from the blood by the liver.

The body simply wants to remain in good shape and will continuously aspire to be in a state of good health.

But how does it do that?

What are the underlying forces that are at work?

The repair processes, the immune response, the proper firing of synapses – all these processes require a well-functioning metabolism.

Without it, nutrients won't be fully absorbed, energy won't be sufficiently produced, and cells won't properly function.

Our body is like a metabolic power station that converts everything we put into it into nutrients and usable energy.

And while this happens on a cellular level, what lies at the heart of this power station is the oven that fires it all up – our digestive system.

But before we get into the Ayurvedic perspective of digestion, I'd like to take a moment and talk about the amazing community of tiny friends without whom none of it would be even possible.

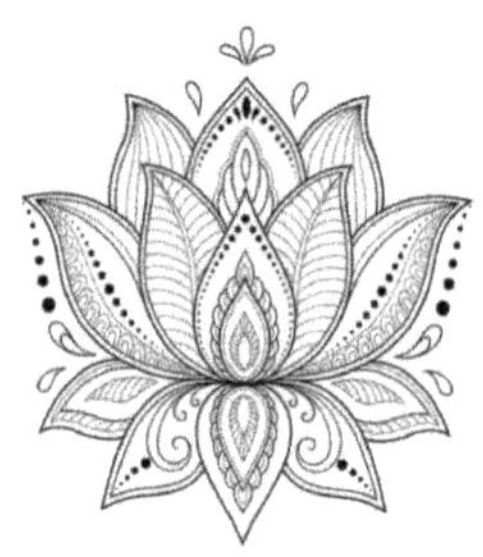

The Microbiome

"We humans are mostly microbes, over 100 trillion
of them. Microbes outnumber our human cells ten to
one. The majority live in our gut, particularly in the
large intestine.
The microbiome is the genetic material of all the
microbes – bacteria, fungi, protozoa, and viruses –
that live on and inside the human body.
The number of genes in all the microbes in one
person's microbiome is 200 times the number of genes
in the human genome. The microbiome may weigh as
much as five pounds."
(dept.washington.edu)

When we are inside our mother's womb, we are pretty much sterile. But when we are born, as we are squeezed through the narrow birth canal, our skin takes on all our mother's bacteria.

These bacteria become the seeds from which our own microbiome and immune system will grow.

This is why babies born via C-section generally have a

slightly weaker immune system and later are more susceptible to developing chronic immune diseases. However, there is much that can be done to counteract this disadvantage.

It takes about two years for the babies' microbiome to be fully formed. It contains bacteria, viruses, fungi, and other organisms, in a ratio that depends both on the mother's internal environment (which forms the seed) and on the child's diet and environment. And there are a lot of them.

The combined cells of all these organisms make up about 90% of the total of our body cells, which means that only 10% of our body cells are actually human – a fact that puts a completely different spin on what being human means.

When we look at the human genome, it becomes even more peculiar – we have about the same genome complexity as a worm (about 21,000 human genes). The full count of genes found in the microbiology of our bodies, however, is 4.4 million. That's about 0.5% of human genes in our bodies and 99.5% of the genome of other organisms.

These organisms come in many shapes and forms. Some of them are harmful and cause acidity and disease if they are not kept in check, some of them are seemingly neutral, and some are extremely beneficial and necessary for our survival. They produce essential vitamins, hormones, and antioxidants, and form a large part of our immune system.

The bacteria in our gut come in a wide variety. Each of them has a preference for different kinds of nutrients.

Our food choices therefore selectively feed and grow colonies of certain types of bacteria and once these bacteria take over, others diminish or even die out.

Bacteria are also capable of communicating with our

brains via the vagus nerve. In this way, they can strongly influence our choices and cravings.

This is partly the reason why, after eating carbohydrate-rich fast food and sugar for some time, we begin to develop a strong longing for these types of food and begin to dislike others, such as vegetables.

The type of bacteria that live in our gut dictate much of our cravings and even have an influence on our moods and behaviours.

Tryptophan, for example, an amino acid that we find in foods like turkey, chicken, eggs, or chia seeds, is converted to serotonin and melanin by the bacteria in our gut. With sufficient amounts of serotonin and melanin in our bodies, we become comfortable and sleepy and can get a good night's rest.

However, if there is an imbalance of gut bacteria, we may not get enough serotonin or melanin, which can eventually lead to insomnia and depression.

Studies show that certain compositions of the microbiome are linked to all kinds of mental health problems.

More and more evidence emerges about the relationship between the constitution of the microbiome and our behaviour.

One particularly interesting study, which was carried out in 2000, highlighted the extent to which microorganisms are capable of altering their host's behaviour.

Toxoplasma gondii is a single-cell parasite that can survive in many species but prefers to live in cats.

When rats were infected with this parasite, not only did they begin to lose their fear of cats, they even became sexually attracted to them. Risking their own death, the rats enabled the parasite to move into their preferred host.

In humans, many such examples are available too. In

autistic children, for example, the constitution and health of the microbiome are directly relatable to the extent of their symptoms.

An imbalance in our microbiome – either inherited or influenced by our environment – can, in many cases, be the first step towards serious disorders and diseases like cancer, Parkinson's, autism, schizophrenia, and more.

These findings are not exactly new.

In the 1800s, a scientist called Ilya Mechnikov discovered, during a cholera epidemic in France, that whether or not a person became sick with cholera depended largely on the consistency of his or her microbiome – some organisms supported the growth of the cholera bacteria while others prevented it.

Unfortunately, his findings were overruled by the inventions of antibiotics, C-sections, pesticides and herbicides, and the microbiome of our gut, as well as that of our soil, deteriorated from then on.

In modern days, stool transplants have become a method of healing the microbiome and its related diseases. Depression has been successfully relieved in this way – through the injection of a healthy person's microbiome.

In acute situations, this may be helpful but from an Ayurvedic perspective, it doesn't really make sense in the long run, unless the treatment is accompanied by a change in the factors that led to the imbalance in the first place.

Eating a one-dimensional diet, overly processed foods, too much sugar or heavy meals, having stress, or a diet that simply doesn't comply with a person's individual constitution can cause an imbalance in the gut.

Each time we take a course of antibiotics, as much as it

can be life-saving, we greatly disturb this balance and it is difficult to build it up again into a balanced diversity. In some cases, there are long-lasting effects.

The Virome

Our microbiome doesn't only consist of bacteria.

As already mentioned, there are billions of organisms living in our gut – mostly bacteria, but many viruses and other microbes too. Each of them has a part to play in our health and the more diversity we can allow, the better.

About 8% of the human genome is derived from viruses. Fossilised and passed on through generations, they have been responsible for much of our evolution, including the development of our placenta. Viruses – as opposed to their bad reputation as the bringers of disease – actually have an important role to play in all of evolution and in our immunity. Without them, we would not exist.

However, a virus is dependent on its environment to multiply. It is kept in check by the complexity of the microbiome and the microbiome, in turn, is influenced (in both positive and negative ways) by the virus. Whether or not a virus takes over and becomes damaging to you, threatening to your body, depends largely on the health and balance of the whole community of microbes.

With this in mind, the best way of disease prevention is not always to try to avoid contact with microbes but to maintain a stable and balanced microbiome.

While on one side, good hygiene is, of course, important to our health, environments that are too sterile, on the other hand, contribute to a lack of diversity in our microbiome and can be the cause of a weak immune system – it's all about finding the right balance.

Stress Factors

However, our microbiome is not only influenced by what we ingest, it is also intimately connected to our nervous system. Not only does our food influence our mood, but our moods influence our digestion.

The microbiome communicates with our nervous system via the vagus nerve, hormones, and immune responses. It directly affects our mental health and behaviour and our ability to cope with stress.

Stress can massively damage the balance of our microbiome, influencing the intake and assimilation of nutrients, our immunity, and our overall health.

Changes in the brain can cause changes in the permeability and secretions in the gut. There are five times as many neurons in the gut as there are in the spinal cord – no wonder it is called the second brain.

The gut-brain axis links emotional and cognitive centres of the brain with gastrointestinal functions.

By feeding the right kind of gut microbes and supporting diversity in our gut environment, we can directly influence our mood and behaviour, mental and physical health, immune system, and hormonal balance.

Immunity

There is only one known case in human history of a person who lived without a microbiome.

David Vetter suffered from severe combined immunodeficiency (SCID) and had absolute no defenses against pathogens. He was born into a plastic bubble and was touched only with plastic gloves until the day he died at age 12.

Antibiotics have saved me from great pain on several occasions and most people I know have depended on them several times during their lives. But taking them does come with a price.

As new studies clearly indicate, the use of antibiotics lowers our immunity significantly, making us much more vulnerable to certain viruses, especially those affecting the lungs.

Children who have been given antibiotics before the age of two are much more likely to develop asthma than those who have not been exposed to them.

Allergies develop mostly in those whose microbiome lacks pathogens and viruses. If you have never had an infection of some sort, you are much more likely to become allergic to something. It is as if your immune system simply needs something to do – if it doesn't, it just attacks something else.

It's not that we should never take antibiotics – sometimes there simply is no other choice – but we do have to carefully weigh up whether their advantage actually outweighs their risks.

What kind of microbiota live in our gut is dependent on our genetic makeup and the micro-biotic "seeds" your mother gave you during birth (Prakruti) as well the ones on the food you eat, the water you drink, the air you breathe, and even the people you live with. These aspects are the ones we can influence and change to enhance our well-being.

The message is clear. Instead of seeing bacteria, and other microbes as enemies to be aggressively fought, we should recognise them as our friends and benefactors, and learn to live with them more harmoniously.

We need to develop a healthy relationship with them and acknowledge the important role they play in our lives.

With only 10 % of human cells and 0.5 % of a human genome, we can clearly see that being human is no special feat - we are, like eveything around us, and interaction of different forms of life. Life isn't even possible without the large, diverse community of microbes, and the sooner we acknowledge this, the better.

When we realise that, with each meal, we aren't just feeding ourselves but our large colonies of microbes, our choices will probably be different.

The better we are as a host, the better they will look after our health.

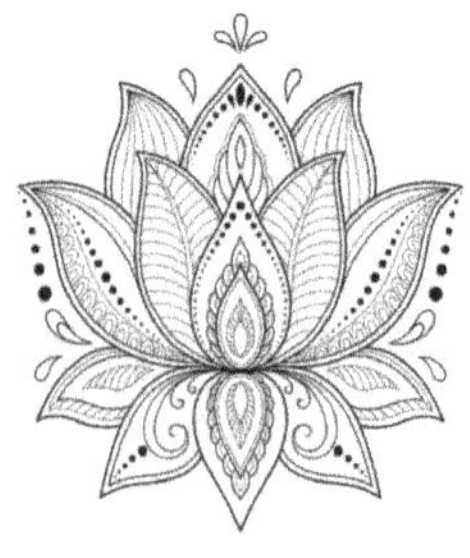

Agni (The Digestive Fire)

The Ayurvedic perspective of digestion is quite simple.

To convert nutrients into energy and building blocks for our tissue cells, we need the energy of fire.

Just like cooking food on a stove, we need to first chop it (chew it well), add water or oil (in the form of our saliva and gastric juices), and then turn up the heat (add energy and enzymic action).

This digestive heat is called Agni.

Agni is the energy that breaks down and transforms food from its original state into usable nutrients and waste. It is the internal fire that activates all metabolic processes.

Agni is everywhere in our bodies. It works through the acidity of hydrochloric acid in the stomach, the enzyme activity in the pancreas, liver, and duodenum; it is present within our endocrine glands, our colon, and in every single cell of our body.

Agni is the internal heat that ignites all physiological processes.

It works on many levels – subtle and gross. Each atom contains Agni, causing chemical reactions and the formation of molecules, and even each thought and emotion must be processed and digested too.

On each of these levels, Agni, the digestive fire, requires different types of fuel and produces different types of energy. Ayurveda distinguishes 40 different types of Agni but, to keep things simple, we will only discuss some of the main ones here.

Jathara Agni (Stomach and Duodenum)

This is the biggest fire in our oven.

It sits in the stomach and is fueled by the food we eat.

Our senses activate it like air fans a fire – we only have to see or smell something delicious and the flames of appetite rise.

When we feel the first pangs of hunger, we know that our stomach is ready to digest.

As soon as the first taste of food touches the tongue, digestive juices begin to flow. Saliva is released and applies initial enzymes to the food, while the stomach's mucus secretions increase to both liquefy the food and protect the stomach lining against the incoming hydrochloric acid.

This stomach acid and the enzymes that are released dissolve the food and break it down into a chyme. This part of the digestive fire – Jathara Agni – is setting the stage for all the following metabolic processes.

It is the fire that cooks the food.

Have you ever tried to light a fire with only large logs and matches? It's not possible. You need well-prepared fuel, stacked properly, and good firelighters or at least dry twigs or paper.

How well you set up the fire, the type of fuel, the kind of kindling, and the quality of your matches all determine how evenly the fire will burn for the next few hours and how much heat it will be able to radiate into the room.

Your appetite is a good indication of Jathara Agni. Those who are blessed with a good appetite generally have a well-functioning Jathara Agni. It means their fireplace is well set up and ready.

Eating without appetite is like throwing big logs onto a tiny, barely flickering flame. We won't be able to properly digest it.

Before we eat a meal, we should be sure to feel hungry. This sounds like an obvious statement, but if we think about it, we often eat without really feeling hungry – maybe we think we should eat, it's time to eat, other people around us are eating, or we may not get the time to eat later. Or maybe we eat out of boredom, emotional longing, or other reasons.

And, of course, it's just as bad to ignore our hunger pangs and let the stomach fire rise up so high that it burns up its environment, bringing about imbalances of Pitta.

If Jathara Agni is steady and strong, food can be optimally pre-digested and prepared for assimilation into the body. Regulating Jathara Agni is one of the first steps in almost any Ayurvedic treatment.

Bhuta Agni (Liver Enzymes)

Bhuta means "essence" or "basic element".

The enzymes in the liver break down the nutrients of the food into these basic elements or molecules, so that they can be transported through the bloodstream. Molecules – from the Ayurvedic perspective – are divided into the five elements of space, air, fire, water and earth, according to their qualities – elements of gas, liquids, solids, energy and the spaces in between.

The liver also filters blood from the heart and from the duodenum and cleanses it from any harmful toxins. These toxins are recycled into bile, which is needed for fat digestion. Some nutrients are also produced and stored in the liver.

The liver is truly a powerhouse of an organ, keeping us healthy and free from toxins, and Bhuta Agni is the force that keeps it working.

Jatru Agni (Thyroid and Thymus Glands)

Jatru Agni refers to both the hormonal activity in the thyroid gland, which regulates our cell metabolism and also to the immune, regulating activities of the thymus gland.

Usually, these two glands would be considered to be a part of the endocrine system instead of the digestive system but Ayurveda has a slightly different view. Because of the important role they play in digestion and in the metabolic functioning of cell tissue, they are just as much a part of the digestive system as they are of the endocrine system.

Jatru Agni produces substances like hormones and white blood cells, which we need for proper digestion, energy metabolism, and immunity. The health of these glands can determine the health of our whole body.

Dhatu Agni (Tissue Cell Metabolism)

After nutrients are sufficiently broken down into small enough particles, or elements, they can be assimilated into the cells.

Not all cells are created equal though; it depends on the type of tissue they make up (Dhatu = tissue).

Ayurveda distinguishes between seven different types of bodily tissue and each of them has its own specific metabolism, structure, and nutritional need.

These metabolic processes are like a chain reaction of nutrient assimilation, production, and waste elimination that happens in a very specific order, much like a row of falling dominos:

1. Rasa Dhatu (blood plasma and white blood cells)
2. Rakta Dhatu (red blood cells)
3. Mamsa Dhatu (muscle tissue)
4. Meda Dhatu (fat tissue)
5. Asthi Dhatu (bones and cartilage)
6. Majja Dhatu (bone marrow, nervous tissue, and connective tissue)
7. Shukra/Arthava Dhatu (male and female reproductive tissue)

The first tissue that is supplied with nutrients is blood plasma (Rasa Dhatu). Rasa Dhatu is the fine nutrient juice that supplies the blood after food is broken down into its elements. These nutrient juices are assimilated into the blood plasma through a Dhatu-specific metabolic process (Rasa Agni) and the leftovers, or eliminations, are then recycled to supply the next tissue – the red blood cells (Rakta Dhatu). The final waste products are then converted into Kapha molecules.

Rakta Agni (red blood cell metabolism) in turn nourishes the red blood cells and produces the nutrients for the next type of tissue cell. Its waste products produce Pitta molecules.

Next comes the nourishment of Mamsa Dhatu, or muscle tissue. The waste products of this metabolism are converted into earwax and nasal and eye discharges, sebum and smegma. Therefore, too much or too little of these substances can tell you a lot about the state of your cell metabolism.

The waste products of Meda Dhatu Agni (fat cell metabolism) produce sweat; the waste products of Asthi Dhatu Agni (bone cell metabolism) produce hair and nails; that of Majja Dhatu Agni (bone marrow and nervous tissue metabolism) produces sebaceous secretions and mucus in the faeces.

The last of the tissue cells to be supplied – the reproductive tissue or Shukra Dhatu – doesn't really produce waste. At this stage, the nutrient supply is so subtle and fine that only a very pure essence is left: Ojas.

Ojas – The Nectar of Life

Ojas is the purest essence of Kapha and is often equated to the immune system. However, it is more than just that. It includes hormones, including oxytocin, serotonin, oestrogen, etc. It includes our sexual fluids and also our cerebrospinal fluids. To have these substances in abundance means to have abundant sexual energy, and the ability to feel joy, love and gratitude in life. It is the substance that enables us to experience the sweetness of life. It is often described as a subtle, honey-like nectar that provides us with the essence of happiness, health and vitality.

The Essences of Abundance

Agni works through increasingly subtle metabolic processes including cell energy metabolism, DNA activity, sense perception, and Doshic balance.

The end product is the pure, subtle essence of our Doshas.

It is the essence of Kapha (Ojas) that protects us from disease and enables us to love and reproduce. Without enough Ojas, we can experience low fertility or libido, low immunity and a lack of joy.

The essence of Pitta – Tejas – is like the essence of fire and light. It gives us intelligence and passion for life and for spiritual growth. We need it to find motivation and a drive to do something in life that will bring us further along in our soul's evolution.

The essence of Vata – Prana – fills us with vitality and grace. Prana is the vital energy that moves through us and enables us to move through life with ease.

If our Agni is strong on all levels, if we have enough Ojas, Tejas and Prana in us, then our energy, intelligence and love will also be strong. Not only will our physiology work more smoothly and without disturbances, our cells are better nourished and our organs better functioning, but our emotional and mental energy will also be clearer.

Our overall feeling of well-being and vitality is directly related to the health and strength of our Agni.

Even the mind has its own Agni. Experiences, too, need to be processed and digested, information stored, and leftovers or unnecessary waste eliminated through creative and emotional expression. These subtle processes are closely connected to the gross mechanics of physical digestion and directly influenced by them. Just like the microbiome influences our brain, the health of our gut, digestion and metabolism influences our mental health. And it all begins with Jathara Agni. We can literally influence the mind through the food we eat.

If we want to live a life of joy and abundance, prevent and heal diseases, disorders and mental imbalances, the best way to begin is by changing our diet and resetting and rebalancing our metabolic system.

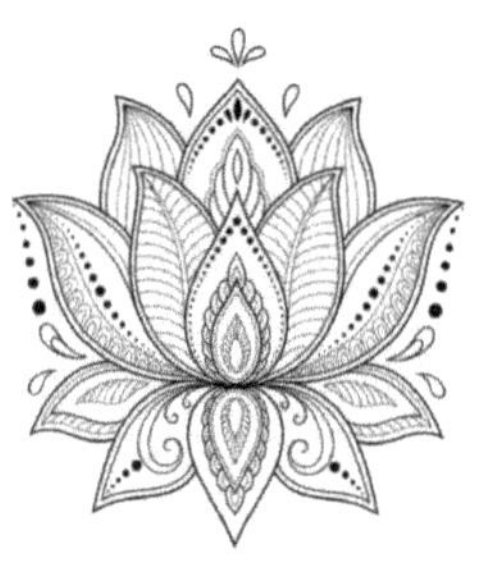

Ama – Toxic Stagnation

If the normal function of Agni is disturbed, the digestive fire becomes too weak, or erratic and unreliable. That means that nutrients won't be properly absorbed and waste products won't fully be eliminated. We may not realise this straightaway, but, over time, it will become apparent. Digestive issues like constipation or diarrhoea, acid reflux or bloating, may show up at first and then, more subtly, the buildup of undigested material in the liver, blood and tissue cells will begin to cause problems such as high blood sugar, cholesterol, calcified arteries, blood clotting, ulcers, uric acid, acetaldehyde (the toxic substance that accumulates in the body when we drink more alcohol than we can metabolise) and other issues of accumulations.

We've probably all experienced a hangover before – it's not pleasant, to say the least. It affects not only our body but also our mind. We might feel depressed, pessimistic and low in energy, our immune system becomes weak, and we lose our confidence and vitality until the toxins have been metabolised and eliminated.

And, of course, it isn't just acetaldehyde that makes us

feel bad. Any undigested substance in the body affects the flow of energy.

Often we are so used to this state that we see it as normal. I have often heard clients say things like, "I didn't even know what it felt like to have real energy for once!"

Waste, from the Ayurvedic perspective, is not toxic. In nature, each creature's waste provides the basis for new growth and life. Anyone who has a garden, knows the value of manure. But waste that is accumulating, and isn't properly absorbed or eliminated, becomes stagnant and toxic.

Toxins, from an Ayurvedic perspective, are food substances or other molecules (also bacteria or viruses), which have not been fully digested and remain stagnant in the body instead of being eliminated as waste or absorbed as nutrients. It is always caused by an insufficient metabolic process.

Whether it is high cholesterol or sugar, acetaldehyde, or a buildup of puss (dead cells and bacteria) in the body, it is sure to affect our health and well-being in some way. Ayurveda refers to this buildup of undigested material as Ama.

We always feel the effect of Ama in our system, even if it's subtle.

The toxic levels in our body don't have to be high to be felt – a subtle lack of energy, an inexplicable pain, a feeling of heaviness, fatigue, and low mood or even depression can be the result of a clogged-up system.

If Ama has been present in the body for a long time, we may have become used to feeling like this and think of it as normal. Doctors don't usually diagnose anything at this early stage and so we often accept this state of being and live on a low level of energy – until we finally change our diet and lifestyle or complete a detox program. Then we probably realise for the first time what it truly means to feel good.

If you are a regular yoga practitioner, or if you work with your body regularly in any other way, you probably feel these subtle buildups more acutely. A daily yoga practice – and this is especially noticeable if it is the same, or a similar sequence each day, as it will provide the constant against which every small change is measured – will feel different depending on what you ate or drank the day before, where you are in your hormone cycle and what kinds of stresses you are experiencing currently.

Your energy levels might be lower, your joints may feel stiffer and your muscles may seem weaker the day after a heavy meal. This can also happen when you are on medication or antibiotics or after a particularly difficult emotional challenge, when, as a response, your digestion slows down. That's why a daily yoga (or other mindful movement) practice is so important – not just for the effect of the asana but for the daily quality time we spend with our body.

If we pay attention to our body and its subtle changes each day, we can notice the body's messages much more clearly and we can react sooner to avoid a more damaging buildup of Ama.

But if we ignore them, it will eventually cause problems.

According to Ayurveda, the presence of Ama in the body, together with an aggravation of Dosha, is the basis for almost all types of disease.

It is clear that when our digestion is not working properly on any level, then nutrients cannot be fully digested and waste products cannot be completely eliminated.

If Jathara Agni is disturbed and Ama collects in the colon (the main seat of Vata and the microbiome), we may feel sluggish and heavy, bloated, gassy, or develop diarrhoea.

If Bhuta Agni in our liver (Ranjaka Pitta) is weak or disturbed and can't keep up with the onslaught of toxins in our system, we might experience immune responses like inflammation or pain.

Too much dryness in the body (Vata) also causes a buildup of Ama, often in the joints, as is the case in rheumatoid arthritis (Ama Vata).

Kapha constitutions, with a naturally low metabolism, are especially prone to a buildup of Ama if they don't adjust their lifestyle accordingly.

Diabetes can develop from an accumulation of glucose and heart disease results from arteries clogged by cholesterol deposits. Eczema, psoriasis, acne, and many more issues result from an accumulation of substances in the body that have not been fully metabolised.

Ama is the cause for most diseases and there are many reasons why it might accumulate in our bodies.

It could be that the digestive process and metabolism are weak and slow and cannot keep up with our intake.

Perhaps we simply eat too much food for our constitution. Even for a strong metabolism, there is a limit. If food is consumed too frequently and not enough time is given for the previous meal to be digested, we are also overtaxing our digestive system. In this way, the body is overwhelmed with different types of demands from the different phases of digestion.

Often we consume foods that are not compatible with our constitution. For instance, a Kapha person whose metabolism is naturally low, who normally has a higher water content and is prone to mucus production will find it difficult to digest heavy, mucus-forming foods like ice-cream, cow's milk, cheese or tofu, and will not be able to convert the concentrated energy of sugar and white flour sufficiently. However, a hot, already acidic Pitta person often can't cope with spicy, acidic, or fried foods or alcohol, which increase the heat, inflammation and acidity in the body even more. Moreover, a light, dry Vata person needs to make an extra effort to stay hydrated and eat substantial, warming, moist and oily foods that nourish their cells.

Furthermore, if we consume too many different types of food or incompatible foods all at once, we can easily weaken our digestive system by diluting Agni. Carbohydrates are digested in a different way to fats and proteins. Dairy needs different types of enzymes to meat or fish or vegetables. Some foods – such as dairy and fruit eaten together – cause fermentation in the body, leading to the formation of toxins, especially in an already weak system.

Unless our digestion is extremely strong, we would do well to keep our meals simple, at least on most days of the week.

And, of course, if we keep eating foods that already contain a lot of toxins or are simply too hard on our digestion – like alcohol, drugs, nicotine, medications, or additives in processed food – Ama will most certainly build up.

If our Agni is strong, food can be digested easily and waste products will be eliminated thoroughly from every cell in our body through our sweat, urine, and faeces. The body will be free of toxins and full of nutrients and form a perfect basis for a disease-free, happy life.

A person with a perfectly strong Agni will be able to eat almost anything they like and digest it without problems.

Even the mind will process things much easier and will more likely be clear and free from toxic thoughts.

But if Agni is weak, neither our mind nor our physiological functions can run smoothly.

Srotamsi – Staying in the Flow

Srotas (plural Srotamsi) is a Sanskrit word meaning "stream", "river", "current" or "channel". It is used to describe the pathways through which nutrients, nervous impulses, waste products, and other substances flow.

Energy in all its forms – be it blood flow, nervous system messages, the pathway of hormones, metabolic pathways, pathways of elimination, etc. – flows in patterns and directions, through membranes, blood vessels, cellular pores or tubes. And just like any other pathway or channel, if it is free of obstacles, its flow is strong and clear.

If your garden hose is blocked and full of chalk and old debris, the water won't flow through it properly. It will just trickle and, eventually, you'll have to buy a new hose.

The channels in our body won't be as easy to replace. It is up to us to look after them to avoid buildup and allow them to clean out from time to time.

Channels are, just like everything else, made of tissue cells, and their health is determined by the health and well-functioning metabolism of these cells.

Ayurveda distinguishes between different types of channels:

Anna Vaha Srotas (The Digestive Tract)

The largest channel in our body is the digestive tract. It includes all the digestive pathways, from the mouth and esophagus through the stomach, duodenum, liver, intestines and the anus.

If the transport of food through this pathway happens in just the right way, everything is fine.

If the flow becomes too much, possibly as an immune response to something bad we've ingested, we might get diarrhoea.

If the flow is too slow, or if it stagnates, a heavy feeling in the stomach, nausea, and constipation is the result. There could also be a problem in the walls of the channel, like gastric ulcers or tumours. And if the direction of the flow is reversed, we vomit. There are many ways in which this channel could be blocked, overflowing or in another way disturbed.

Prana Vaha Srotas (The Respiratory System)

From breathing in and out to oxygenation of blood cells, Prana Vaha Srotas is the pathway of Prana – the life force we take in with our breath. It is more than just oxygen; it is the subtle essence of Vata, the energy of space and air that gives our body the ability to move and function. Without Prana, the heart would not beat, the diaphragm would not contract, our nervous system would not function and our organs would shut down.

Prana is the vital energy responsible for all movements in our body and, therefore, for life itself. It also has a pathway that has to be clear of obstructions like mucus buildup or toxins from smoking or pollution, or blocked receptors in our nerve cells.

Udaka Vaha Srotas (The Water Pathway)

Our bodies consist mostly of water.

When we drink, even water has to be digested, cleansed, and made available to the tissue cells. In fact, drinking water alone does not ensure proper cell hydration.

Everywhere in the body, there are glands that secrete water in its different forms and stages of digestion.

All these secretions are really one flow, one pathway of water.

Ayurveda sets the beginning stages of the cycle in the pancreas, where enzyme-rich water is released, and in the soft palate, which produces saliva. It continues in the tongue, the choroid plexuses in the brain that secretes cerebrospinal fluid, the mucus membrane in the GI tract, the kidneys, and the sweat glands. When these pathways are blocked, the pores of the cells are obstructed or dried out. Sometimes the cell walls are not elastic enough, which means that water won't reach the cell's inner organelles, or it may become retained in the wrong places. Additionally, if we block our skin pores with harsh deodorants, preventing sweating, then toxins won't be eliminated properly anymore.

Dhatu Srotamsi (The Metabolic Pathways of the Tissues)

The way the tissue cells are supplied with nutrition also happens along very specific pathways.

We've talked about the seven bodily tissues (Dhatus) already.

When food is broken down into its basic components, the first tissue to be supplied is Rasa Dhatu – blood plasma and lymph. After it is metabolised in these cells, the remaining products are carried into the next tissue: Rakta Dhatu, or red blood cells. From here, the metabolites are moved into muscle tissue cells (Mamsa Dhatu), fat cells (Meda Dhatu), bone tissue (Asthi Dhatu), bone marrow and nervous tissue cells (Majja Dhatu) and, finally, reproductive tissue cells – Shukra Dhatu (male) and Arthava Dhatu (female).

If any of these subtle pathways, including the pores in each cell, are not functioning properly or are blocked with Ama, nutrients cannot fully be metabolised by the cell and it, despite us eating sufficiently, might be starved of nutrition.

And as the tissue cell pathways are really a chain reaction of metabolic activities, if there is a blockage in one of the Dhatu Srotas, all remaining tissues will be affected too.

It is quite possible that one part of the body may be over-nourished while another doesn't get enough nutrition.

We can often see that in people who suffer from obesity.

Channels of Elimination

As a result of our metabolic pathways, waste is eliminated from the cells, the blood, and the digestive tract and carried out of the body through sweat (Sweda Vaha Srotas), urine (Mutra Vaha Srotas) and faeces (Purisha Vaha Srotas).

It is already clear that should these channels be obstructed or dysfunctional in in any way, wastes cannot be properly eliminated and toxins have a greater chance to accumulate in the body.

Women also have two extra channels:

Rajah Vaha Srotas (The Menstrual Channel)

If the pathways of menstruation are not clear and well functioning, many issues, from PMS to polycystic ovaries, can develop. Nowadays there are many options to "ease" our cycle by taking hormones that can completely block the flow of menstrual blood. We often talk about our menstruation in derogatory terms and with annoyance, as if it is nothing but an inconvenience. But our menstruation is an important way of cleansing the system before potential new life moves in. We rid ourselves of not only physiological toxins but also emotional ones. We may at times feel irrationally sad or angry about something we can't even quite remember. This is our way of clearing unfinished business from our unconscious mind, so that it doesn't fester in our cells and DNA. It is an extraordinary function we can be grateful for.

Stanya Vaha Srotas (The Lactation Channel)

Some of you may have experienced a blocked milk duct. It is very unpleasant and can quickly develop into mastitis – an infection of these ducts, which can be extremely painful for the woman. Fortunately, this can be remedied by natural medicines with relative ease.

Mano Vaha Srotas (The Channel of the Mind)

The mind is also considered a channel. Information is absorbed and processed, and its unused waste products are eliminated through voice and creative expression.

Our mind is not separate from our body. Through our heart, our senses, and our nervous and endocrine systems, all our experiences influence our physiology – and changes in our physiology have, through the same pathways, an effect on our mood and mental health. What we experience and how we process it affects our physical health and what we eat; how we digest it affects our mental health.

It is important to keep in mind that to be fully healthy, the digestive processes of the mind cannot be ignored.

As they are more subtle, they often lay the basis for our physical state and no healing is complete without addressing issues of the mind.

Our mind also has its own Prakruti – we are all different and our minds work in different ways.

The Vedic philosophy of Samkhya – which provides the basis for Ayurveda – describes the states of mind through the Gunas Sattva, Rajas and Tamas.

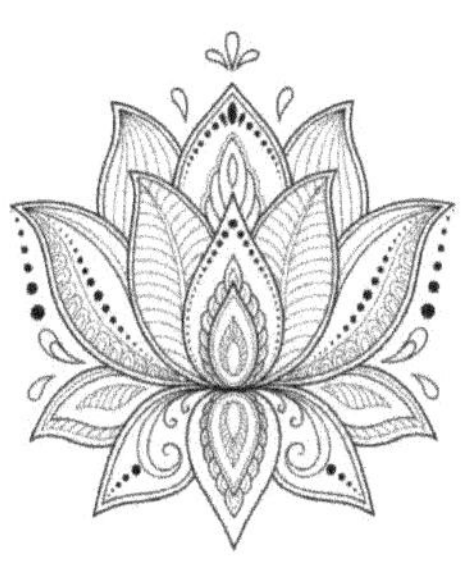

The Gunas of the Mind

Sattva

A sattvic mind is a mind that is in a state of joy, love, bliss and true contentment. We experience this state when we are deep in meditation or in a creative flow, or when we are feeling in love. It is a mind that can flow freely without blockages and is thus completely absorbed by the present moment. It is in balance with the world, in a state of peace. Like a flower in bloom that gives off fragrance and beauty, or like a full moon that radiates light, the sattvic mind radiates light in the form of inspiration. A sattvic mind inspires its surroundings without wanting to control them. It is aware that it is a part of the universal flow – not separate, but a microcosmic expression of the whole universe. It feels a sense of belonging and contentment. This is a state most of us know from brief moments of happiness, in deep immersion in any creative, spiritual, emotional or intellectual activity we truly enjoy.

When we are one with ourselves, without the desire to be different, when we can show ourselves to the world as we really are, without fear of rejection or exclusion, without expectations, without envy, then we are in a sattvic state.

Sattva is always relative to rajas and tamas, which means that when rajas and tamas are in balance in our lives, sattva automatically dominates. For example, if we find a healthy balance between productivity and movement (rajas) and sleep and relaxation (tamas), then our mind will be optimally inspired.

Rajas

A rajasic mind is no longer completely satisfied. It is no longer absorbed by the here and now, but is drawn to the future. It is full of desire for a conscious or unconscious goal. It is agitated, preoccupied, thinking of what is yet to be done or of what it would like to acquire. It wishes for something it does not have at this moment, bringing it away from a state of present moment awareness and therefore away from a state of happiness, bliss and contentment. It tries to achieve something, criticises, feels emotions like anger, excitement, passion or desire.

Such a state is not always bad – we are all in a rajasic state for the most part of the day. Without that state, we wouldn't be productive. It is only through the desire of Rajas that we evolve as human beings. It is a state we need to achieve anything – but it is also a state we need to be very careful with, because it can easily draw us into a world of unsatisfied emotions, overstimulation, lust, anger and stress.

Dynamic movement and productive work is an important part of our lives. And that is exactly what we need as human beings. If we lack the feeling of productivity in life, we soon feel useless. Life then seems to make little sense and we easily fall into depression (tamas). But productivity must inspire us (sattva) so that we can live it sustainably.

Rajasic physical exercise – sports, dynamic yoga, workouts – are also important for our health and for preventing depression and many physical diseases.

Tamas

A tamasic mind lives in the past. It is a dull mind that does not move forward or upward, but instead pulls us downward in a heavy and sluggish way. We all experience a tamasic state of mind when we are asleep or feeling tired, or when we feel the heaviness of pessimistic thoughts and difficult memories. But we also need this state of mind at times, to rest and regenerate, to balance too much rajas. Only when it takes over and begins to dominate our mind, we may face many challenges – depression, addiction, selfishness, greed, laziness, dullness and also disease. But before we can achieve a sattvic state of mind, we have to first go through Rajas. To get out of an overly tamasic state, we need exercise and movement ignite a desire in us that motivates us and fills us with incentive and energy to bring us out of the heaviness again. Becoming aware of our condition in the first place is the first step. The way out of depression or suppressed anger is to consciously feel the emotion, only then can we let it go. With such emotions, it is as if they were a small child seeking attention: the child only stops whining when it has been given the feeling of being heard. Even if it doesn't ultimately get what it wants, as long as it feels acknowledged and loved, it can eventually relax.

It is the same with our feelings. We first have to listen to ourselves, acknowledge and respect who we are in this moment, with all our shadows and scars. Only then can we relax, calm down and see clearly. And in this clear vision, it is much easier to find motivation again and, through the balance of rajas and tamas, eventually return to the desired sattvic state.

To go from a tamasic state of laziness, depression and inertia to a daily yoga and meditation practice is too big a step for most. We need to take smaller steps. It is best to do what comes easily to us first. Just one minute of meditation, one asana a day can be enough to make a start. If that one minute feels good, we can then extend it to two minutes. One asana becomes five. In this way, we can grow beyond our own shadow without overextending ourselves.

Prakruti and Our Mental State

In order to even take these first steps, we must first acknowledge the present moment and accept whatever state we are in right now.

If we ignore our own individual nature by trying to adapt to the expectations of others, we will never be truly happy. We will most likely be constantly dissatisfied with ourselves and our surroundings. We may develop more and more of an inner belief that we are not good enough. Over time, we may separate ourselves more and more from our community, family or culture because we feel that we just don't really belong.

Especially for children who are building up their beliefs and whose outlook and self-image are still extremely impressionable, it is important that they feel respected and loved exactly as they are.

A Vata child, for example, will naturally tend to seek independence and freedom – both physically and mentally. Vata children are born rebels and creative free thinkers. A Vata child cannot stand injustice or interference with its freedom of movement. If a Vata child has to sit still for hours at school, this inevitably leads to feelings of restlessness, anxiety and resistance. Often these days, natural Vata children are marked with labels such as ADHD simply because they cannot meet the standard of our current schooling methods. Vata children are also often highly sensitive. Experiences that other siblings might take with a pinch of salt could have a much more traumatic effect on a Vata child.

Kapha children, on the other hand, are naturally calmer and slower in their movements, both physically and mentally. They learn more slowly and need more sensory stimulation and emotional involvement to do so, but they have a great memory and retain what they do learn very well. If you put such a child in a social environment where speed and competition are predominant, they can easily feel inadequate and lose self-esteem. Kapha children are generally loving, helpful and cuddly and need a lot of rest and time for daydreaming. They have great social intelligence, but if they are not respected in their individuality, their self-esteem will suffer and it will be difficult for them to develop their amazing potential.

A Pitta child, on the other hand, needs a sense of challenge. If a Pitta child is expected to follow a curriculum that does not do justice to his or her abilities, boredom and frustration will arise. The frustration will easily turn the fire of Pitta into anger, which will then surface elsewhere, depending on personality. A Pitta child, more than others, needs a way to focus all of its concentrated energy. It needs challenge and the feeling of achievement. Their innate abilities to organise or to be leaders must somehow be able to be used in a positive way, otherwise the fire that naturally burns within them easily becomes a destructive blaze.

Whether or not we are respected as children is crucial to our later life. All these early experiences form the basis for what we identify with later as adults, what beliefs we develop and how we understand the world around us.

About 90% of our mental and emotional activities take place in our subconscious mind. It might be hard to imagine, but this means, of course, that we are not consciously aware of most of our thoughts and feelings.

But we can imagine how much of our behaviour is controlled by these unconscious, conditioned thoughts and feelings that we have accumulated over the course of our lives.

Unconscious conditioning and old traumas that we have experienced or even inherited through our DNA determine how we experience the world today.

And most – if not all – traumatic experiences have something to do with not being seen, accepted or loved as we really are. Many, perhaps all, trauma experiences are based on experiences that have taught us that we will be rejected if we show ourselves as we really are.

So becoming aware of what we actually feel in each moment, what we really want in life and who we really are – accepting and respecting our own nature, including all wounds and shadows – is a crucial step for us that we cannot avoid if we want to achieve real mental and physical health.

Authenticity is an absolute prerequisite for anyone hoping for success in their spiritual development.

Enlightenment means shining the light of consciousness on the darker, unconscious sides of our mind. Enlightenment is nothing more than freeing ourselves from all of our unconscious conditioning so that we can see the world as it really is, rather than through the subjective filters we have created for ourselves.

The more we can erase old, unconsciously programmed behaviour and thought patterns from our mind, the clearer we will be able to see things and the less threatening the world will seem. We will be able to see the beauty and perfection of the world in everything and everyone around us and make decisions based on inner wisdom rather than out of compulsion.

By living truthfully according to our own nature, we can experience a sense of freedom, joy and belonging.

With each liberation from an old belief, we release a lot of energy that was previously blocked by it. This energy can then be used to heal ourselves from mental or physical imbalances and to live out our true potential in this world with all its infinite possibilities.

From a Vedic perspective, this is exactly why we are here in the first place – to go on a journey of enlightenment. Even our ancient myths and fairy tales tell of nothing else:

life is a hero's journey. In the old fairy tales and legends, the respective hero represents the masculine principle (Purusha), an archetype of consciousness that is searching for its missing half (Prakruti). This feminine principle stands for our individual nature, our physical and mental constitution. To reunite the two, we must first leave our current comfort zone to enter another world – the underworld, or the world of the unconscious mind. Here, we have to find our way across a slippery and unknown path and eventually face our inner demons, in the form of our own shadows. Once we have managed to defeat these demons (usually with the help of magical weapons), we can unearth the treasures (energy) they have been guarding. Only then can we reunite our split duality, marry the feminine and masculine in us and integrate what was previously lost in embodied change, to finally become confident and empowered kings and queens of our own lives.

In reality, there are many such magical weapons available to us – yoga, pranayama, meditation, a good diet and many more methods that provide us with the strength we need to rid ourselves of mental and physical toxins.

Perhaps at first it seems impossible for us to be absolutely free of any such toxicity.

And off course, there is always a certain amount of Ama present in body and mind and, as I said, the presence alone is nothing bad – on the contrary, a little healthy stress contributes to our psychological development after all. That's why it wouldn't be helpful to obsessively want to avoid all toxins and to separate ourselves too much from our environment in the process. Just like avoiding all bacteria in our environment would lead to nothing but a deprived immune system that would, in the end, also contribute to even more disease.

The most important thing is always awareness.

Being aware of what we feel, think and do, so that over time we can learn to distinguish which of our desires come from the heart (the seat of the soul) and which come from our ego (our unconscious beliefs) because both often want quite the opposite. The ego always craves a feeling of security, while the soul wants transformation.

In the end, the soul always wins. But the journey can be long and arduous, if we keep ignoring the soul's needs.

The cosmic intelligence that lives in our body, will communicate these needs to us in the form of outcries of pain and frustration, stiffness or physical symptoms. The unconscious mind will keep recreating unpleasant situations for us that eventually will force us to leave our comfort zone and begin this journey of transformation.

It would be good for us to acknowledge that we ourselves have the power over our destiny. Every moment in our lives offers an opportunity to choose between the soul or the ego – what we ultimately do is up to us alone.

Ojas – More Than Just Immunity

When food is digested fully and all seven bodily tissues are nourished adequately, what remains, in the end, is a biological essence called Ojas.

It is the essence of the water elements of our food and all our bodily tissues. We can imagine it as the life-giving essence of primal water. It nourishes us on a subtle level and provides the basis for our health and well-being. It gives us not only immunity, but also life, vitality, and sensuality. It creates our sex hormones and cerebrospinal fluid. We are all born with a certain amount of this life-giving essence stored in the heart, which we call Paramojas – the Ojas that was there before. Paramojas is irreplaceable. When it is used up, we die. But out of it, we can create Aparamojas – the type of Ojas that is useable and renewable. It is a little bit like having a certain amount of money in the bank. Once it is used up, it is gone but from this money we can draw smaller amounts, and if we use them wisely, we can even increase them through investments. In that way, we can extend our lifespan and increase our well-being quite significantly.

Ojas is the essence of all the pure qualities of Kapha when it is in balance.

People with good Ojas often have a well-developed libido and an ability to truly enjoy life. They are attracted to other people and tend to see the best in them. They love life and recognise its beauty everywhere. They also seem particularly attractive to others, not only because of their well-nourished looks but because of the love they exude. Their constitution is strong – they are not only immune to many infections but also towards many stresses of life.

When we age and enter the Vata phase of our life, our Ojas slowly begins to dry out – production of our sex hormones decreases, our hair begins to thin and our skin dries out and wrinkles. We also become more vulnerable to infections and degenerative diseases.

Ojas is the first of the subtle essences. It nourishes other life-giving energies – Tejas and Prana – and to increase and protect it is one of the main goals of many yogic practices.

Tejas – The Light of Inspiration

Tejas is the essence of fire and that of a balanced Pitta Dosha. It is the subtle essence of our metabolism, the innate intelligence of each of our cells, our physiological functions, and our brain.

It is the internal light that shines through us and makes our minds sharp and focused. It enhances our senses and perception and makes our eyes shine with alertness and understanding.

People who possess a lot of Tejas often look like they are glowing from the inside. They have a passion and a zest for life. They follow their deepest desires, which lead them along an authentic path through life, and they have an ability to fully embrace their experiences. They are motivated and courageous people who don't shy away from obstacles. They have a great capacity to achieve true success in whatever they set out to do as long as it is coming from their own, inner truth.

Their digestion of both food and emotional/mental experiences is usually excellent.

But Tejas, just like Ojas, can be depleted. If we overuse our intelligence in a one-directional way, if we overtax our digestive system, or if we become overly competitive workaholics, losing the connection to our own authentic self, the inner glow may soon burn itself out.

Prana – Vitality of Life

Prana – the pure essence of balanced Vata – is the life force that is responsible for all movement, including the beating of our hearts, our breath, and the firing of synapses in our brain. Without movement, there is no life, no energy, no vitality.

All of life is a dance, in which the basic qualities of life – the Gunas – react to each other, trying to reach a state of balance.

When our breath stops, our hearts will stop too and when stillness enters the body, our life will come to an end.

But too much movement also creates problems. If our heart beats uncontrollably fast, if we hyperventilate, or if our nervous system breaks down due to an overload of information, we are also in trouble.

All of life's movement is about balance.

It is about finding a balance between activity and rest, between nourishment and detoxification, between the mind and the senses, passion and surrender.

If we can maintain this balance by remaining in harmony with our inner and outer world, we are, like a dancer in synchronicity with the music, moving through life with grace.

People with a lot of Prana are full of vitality. Their bodily functions and their minds work smoothly, and they don't tire easily. Playful and creative, they actively move through life, radiant, vibrant and graceful. They can handle change with ease.

Ojas, Tejas and Prana can be increased and protected firstly though a healthy diet. Food that is natural and whole – such as fresh vegetables, grains, pulses and fruit that are gently cooked and have not been processed, canned or frozen – can be digested easily and therefore supports the production of Ojas in our body. In addition, it contains its own vital essences, which we ingest and add to our own.

Secondly, if we can live a lifestyle in harmony with the natural energies around us, we can access them and powerfully increase our own.

That means sleeping when it is dark and waking at first light, so that we can get the most amount of sunlight. It means eating our biggest meal at midday, when the energies of fire in the atmosphere are at their strongest, just like our own, so that we can make the most of our digestion. And it means eating according to our climate and seasons and according to our own constitution.

The Dance of Life

Nothing in life is permanent.

Like every other manifestation in the universe, our human bodies are designed to change – they grow, move, are subject to constant internal transformation and, eventually, they disintegrate back into the matrix of nature to nourish new forms of life.

From an Ayurvedic perspective, death is not the end, but simply part of an eternal fluctuation. Just like a foetus who is about to be born must feel as if it is about to die – its world, as it knows it, is ending and it is in pain and fear as it moves through the birth canal before it sees the "light at the end of the tunnel". In truth, it is only the beginning of something new.

The Vedic perspective differs from our western one in that death is not the end of life. Life itself is eternal; it simply changes form. The body is simply shed, like a snake sheds its skin, in order to manifest a new one that is more in line with our soul's evolutionary state. We suffer only because of our innate instinct to desperately grasp onto life as we know it but if we were able to let go easily, we would quite likely see death simply as another transformation – an expansion of our soul into wider dimensions.

In any case, none of us will be able to avoid it, nor should we want to. Each night, we go to sleep and each morning, we wake up refreshed and rejuvenated. It wouldn't occur to us to want to extend one day forever, avoiding its end to never go to sleep because we trust that we will wake up again. If we had the same faith, that same certainty of being reborn into a new life, we might loose a little of our fear of death.

A certain amount of fear is of course natural to the human condition – we all feel it to some extent. But to let the fear of death extend into a fear of anything unknown, and to let it guide our behaviour and experience of life – and love – is neither desirable nor necessary.

Life is not something that happens to us. It is something we create, even if the process of creation happens on a mostly unconscious level.

Death is nothing bad – it is a necessary renewal of life.

We are like all of nature around us. We decay and we renew and whatever seeds are lodged underneath the surface of the soil will sprout and grow and bear fruit during the next season.

This is Karma. The subtle, unconscious conditionings – both good or bad – are the seeds that determine what kind of life we will manifest in the future.

Life as we know it is governed by duality. There is no life without death, no death without birth. For us to truly understand something, we have to also understand its dual opposite. If we want to understand joy, we have to have known suffering before.

Stress, too, isn't always something bad – it is necessary in order to create change and evolution. Stress is a natural part of the human experience, and it is important for us to experience it as long as it isn't greater than our capacity to handle it.

We all know that (within a certain limit, of course) the more pathogens our immune system encounters, the stronger it will be.

We know that avoiding pathogens completely is not only impossible but doesn't make any sense, as we would take away our immune system's very reason for existence, and with nothing else to do, it will begin to attack other substances from the food we eat to our own tissue cells.

We also know that the more diverse our microbiome, the healthier it is. And we know that in the long run, viruses are not all bad – like everything in existence, they too have a purpose and a role to play in contributing to the evolution of our genetic makeup.

Stress and trauma are certainly a challenge for us. But without any kind of challenge, we would not grow. We need a certain amount of stress in our lives to become stronger and healthier people.

Yet again, it is all about the balance, and our capacity to process and digest our experiences and eliminate their waste. Yet again, it all comes down to the strength and functioning of our mental and physical Agni.

The Body as a Messenger of the Soul

There is so much we can do to support the metabolic functions of our body and keep our Doshas in balance.

Once we understand the Ayurvedic view of the human body and its digestive processes, we know exactly what can be done to support the body's natural functions.

The state of our health is largely up to us and what we decide to do.

Sometimes I hear someone say, "But we have to have a little fun in life too!"

Yes, I totally agree. A life without fun and joy is nothing desirable – the Vedic scriptures also say that.

But I don't want to have just "a little" fun and then pay for it later with a lot of suffering. On the contrary. I want to enjoy life deeply and completely; I want to experience every moment consciously and feel the joy and fun in all situations.

And this also includes experiencing and enjoying my own body intensely.

I compare our relationship with our body to a relationship between mother and child.

As a mother, I love my children with great passion. I have enjoyed every stage of their lives, from infancy into adulthood, even the difficult periods of adolescence. Even though I have been desperate at times, I do not regret any of the challenges that came with it – and there were many.

I love my children just as they are.

I love them without expecting them to be perfect. I love them not only when they are beautiful, bring home good grades or dutifully do everything I ask them to do. I love them as unconditionally as a human being can.

And I have always had a lot of fun with them.

In fact, I associate the time I have spent with my children with much more fun and joy than any alcohol-soaked party I had during my youth. Taking care of them, cooking for them, playing games with them, telling stories, dancing and travelling with them, and helping them when they are in need makes my heart overflow with love and for me there is nothing more beautiful and joyful than feeling deep love and connection.

And that's how I see my relationship with my body.

Developing a loving relationship with the body and respecting it is much more fun than ignoring or exploiting it. Such a relationship forms the basis for health, well-being and joy in life.

If I constantly ignore my body and its messages, I cannot expect to really know it or feel comfortable in it.

In my opinion, one of the most important things we can do is to cultivate a deep love for and respect of our own bodies. Our body is absolutely perfect just the way it is. Every cell in it works tirelessly to keep us in balance. The body has no ego. It never lies. It is divine, cosmic intelligence.

Our body is the best and most honest friend we have in life.

Even if we need to make a change – lose weight or overcome a health problem – we should do it out of love, not out of fear or social pressure. That way, the process will come much more natural and easy to us.

If we simply become more familiar with our body, take some time to get to know its individual qualities without judgement, and let go of conditioned expectations, everything else will follow much more easily. The body really is a messenger of our soul. All symptoms, every little discomfort, pain or illness, tells us something about the state of our soul.

However, the soul and the ego usually want different

things. The soul wants transformation, development and awareness, the ego wants security and a well known routine. And this discrepancy can then easily lead to suffering: We want to eat healthier, but our subconscious holds on too tightly to old habits.

The more we learn to respect and love our bodies, the more we reconnect with our original nature and then a healthy, balanced lifestyle will come quite naturally to us.

Of course, if there is an urgent health problem, it is important to see a doctor instead of experimenting on yourself. A doctor will be able to diagnose the problem and give advice aimed at stopping the symptoms. This can be important if the symptoms are putting us at risk.

An Ayurvedically trained therapist can additionally trace the origin of the problem back to its origin, so that the cause can be eliminated. Then an individual treatment plan can be created that, in addition to treating the symptoms, supports the body in its self-healing and detoxification processes.

Reversing a disease completely is more common than many people might think, but of course it is not always possible. It depends on how serious the problem is and how far it has progressed. However, the earlier we recognise the first signs, the sooner we can do something about it.

Again, I liken this to our children. If I keep watching my child's development and react to its needs when he or she is young, I can prevent problems for her or him later in life, which might be difficult to reverse otherwise, both on a physical and on a mental level.

It is, of course, best not to let it get that far in the first place.

The responsibility for preventing disease is in our own hands.

From an Ayurvedic point of view, the cause of the vast majority of diseases is prajnaparadha – a "crime against wisdom".

How "wise" we actually behave is up to us.

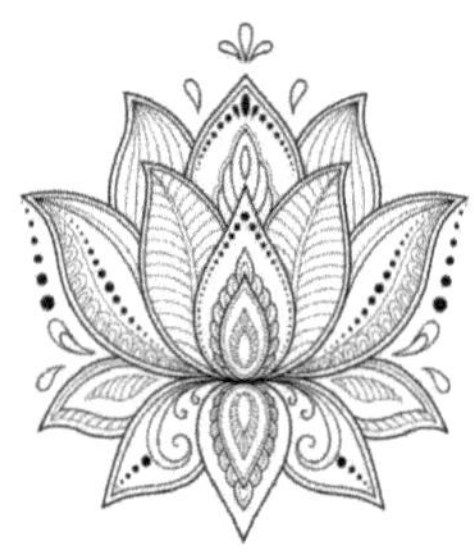

Part 3
Recipes & Advice

Radical Self Love

The first step towards greater health and happiness is to assess the present moment. What is my actual true nature, my genetic constitution and what is the state my body and mind are in right now? To understand ourselves on all levels – physically, emotionally, mentally and spiritually – takes time and practice.

This "practice" can consist of a daily yoga practice, for example.

Yoga, when we place our awareness on our breath and listen to the subtle sensations in our body, teaches us the habit of paying attention to what is going on even on a cellular level. When we spend a certain amount of quality time every day with our body – even if it is only a few minutes – in full awareness of all its subtle changes, we learn to listen. We understand the effect a heavy meal the night before has on our energy levels. We learn to appreciate the monthly cycles and their effect on our strength, flexibility and mental state. And gradually we become more and more fine-tuned towards the messages our body is trying to convey.

Slowly, this heightened awareness may spill over into our

daily lives and we find it easier to pay attention to how we feel after a certain meal or activity. This direct perception tells us much more than any quiz or book ever could and we should listen to it.

Even if you don't have a diagnosed gluten intolerance, if you feel bloated or heavy after eating bread, just cut down on it. Your body's messages are clear. Don't second-guess them. This is how we learn to listen and to make ourselves a priority. Because we are worth it!

We just need to be careful not to get overly obsessive about our eating habits. To become uptight and stressed, or judgmental about the perception of others isn't conducive to a state of balance either. It is best is to stay in a state of relaxed awareness and compassion with oneself and everyone around us.

An Ayurvedic practitioner will be able to analyse your Vikruti and Prakruti through thorough questioning and observation of your physical signs. This is the best way if you really want to get to the bottom of a disorder you are suffering from.

But to help you reflect a little bit more by yourself and get an overall picture, I've prepared a quiz for you.

Simply answer the questions and award yourself one point for each P (Pitta), K (Kapha) and V (Vata).

When you have counted up your answers, you might see one Dosha being clearly dominant over the others. Or maybe you have an equal mix of two. All Doshas can, of course, be aggravated at the same time but you have to figure out which one is the most pressing to deal with first. If you are suffering from a disorder like constant diarrhoea, or some inflammatory disease that causes you suffering, then look at the answers here first. The imbalance that is most pressing and causes most pain or suffering will need to be treated first.

And, of course, always keep in mind that taking a quiz is not a substitute for an actual consultation with a trained practitioner.

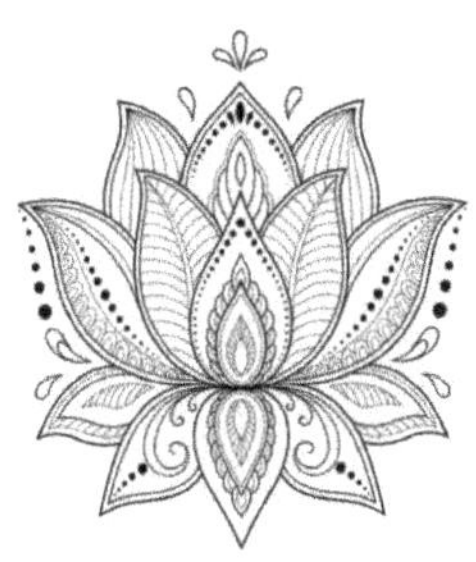

Dosha Quiz

Your Physical Constitution

1. Are you usually hungry in the morning?

P   yes

K   no

V   not sure/sometimes

2. How many meals do you eat a day?

P   3 regular meals a day; sometimes a snack.

K   1-3 meals a day. You actually get by with very little, but eat out of habit or because you love the taste.

V   Several small meals/snacks a day; you sometimes forget to eat.

3. You eat mainly because:

P   you are hungry

K   out of habit/because of the taste

V   because you need the energy

4. Sometimes you experience:

P   heartburn, stomach ulcers, diarrhoea.

K   tiredness, bloating, slow bowel movement

V   flatulence, pain, constipation

5. Your figure is rather:

P   average/athletic

K   curvy/voluminous/thick-boned

V   thin/light/above-average height or weight

6. You tend to:

P   maintain an even weight

K   gain weight easily

V   lose weight easily

7. When you get sick, it is usually:

P   something inflammatory/fever, allergies, infections or digestive problems.

K   mucus buildup, high blood sugar/cholesterol or respiratory problems

V   pain/psychological problems/fatigue or deficiencies

8. Your bowel movements are:

P   light and regular/more than once a day, soft

K   regular/once a day or less, bulky

V   more irregular, small, dry pieces

9. You often feel:

P   hot, sweaty, too warm

K   cold, clammy

V   cold hands or feet

10. Your blood pressure tends to be:
P   high
K   low
V   variable

11. Your natural hair is:
P   blonde/light/red, wavy, fine or prematurely greying
K   dark, thick, lush or curly
V   thin, dry, frizzy, tight curls, falling out

12. Your tongue is:
P   reddish/pink in colour, fairly clean or with a greenish coating
K   thick and large, with a white coating
V   small or thin, with cracks in the middle or on the back

13. Your skin is:
P   fair/rosy, prone to acne, sunburn/rashes or freckled
K   smooth, oily/large-pored, not particularly sensitive
V   dry, scaly, premature wrinkles, sensitive, comparatively dark

14. Your eyes are:
P   bright, luminous, highly pigmented or sensitive to light
K   large, shiny, loving look, thick eyelashes/eyebrows
V   small, dry, restless look, thin eyelashes/eyebrows

15 Your body hair is rather:
P   medium, light
K   dark or dense, lots of body hair
V   thin, curly, fine

16. Your muscle strength/endurance is:

P   average, athletic

K   strong, enduring, lots of power, good for slow, leisurely sports

V   rather weak, short, strong bursts of energy, well suited for fast-paced sports

17. Your voice is:

P   clear, with precise articulation

K   warm, soft, pleasant voice, good singing voice

V   particularly high or low, you talk more or less than average, irregular, imprecise

18. Your teeth are:

P   average, yellowish

K   large, firm, white teeth

V   small, irregular teeth, caries, weak bite

19. Your nails are:

P   round, rosy, soft

K   strong, smooth, shiny, large

V   brittle, irregular, small, grooves

20. Your tongue is:

P   reddish, red spots, blood blisters, medium in size.

K   thick, swollen, lots of white coating

V   many lines, irregular, deep teeth marks on the sides

So much for your physical constitution.
Now answer a few more questions about your psychological constitution:

Your Psychological Constitution

Social life

V   Many acquaintances, frequently changing friends, unreliable, flighty

P   Inspiring, meaningful friendships, useful social networks

K   Few, but very close, long-lasting friendships, loyal

Creativity

V   Very creative, many ideas but not enough patience to realise them

P   Planned projects, implements ideas well, organised

K   Traditional or practical creativity (cooking/baking, decorating, sewing, pottery etc.)

Intelligence

V   Grasps quickly and also forgets quickly, learns well by listening, creative intelligence

P   Focused, grasps quickly and retains well, visual learning, analytical intelligence

K   Grasps slowly but does not forget. Learns best through personal experience and feelings. Emotional intelligence

Family dynamics

V   Likes to be independent, needs a lot of freedom, is often the outsider of the family, more sensitive than others, often moves further away from the family

P   Likes to take responsibility, knows what is best for everyone, likes to organise, critical and argumentative, generous

K   Maternal, keeps the family together, emotional, traditional values, cares and worries about everyone

Emotions

V   Sensitive, fluctuating emotions, frequent ups and downs, reacts quickly, anxious, worrying, nervous

P   Must have everything under control, critical, gets angry or irritated, passionate, judgmental

K   Stable, can take a lot, martyr, rarely reacts angrily (but when they do, it's for a long time), loving and caring, manipulative, clingy, depressive

Stress management

V   Reacts quickly to stress, sensitive nervous system, nervous, quickly overwhelmed, quickly worried, flight response

P   Reacts well to stress but tends to burn-out, easily irritated by others, perfectionist and impatient, takes the lead in stressful situations, fight response

K   Strong nervous system, patient, can take a lot, stays calm in stressful situations, freeze response

In general, you can say that all the things you can answer in a positive way – the positive, healthy qualities of Vata, Pitta or Kapha – belong to your individual Prakruti and the more negative, unbalanced ones to your Vikruti.

If in doubt, just do the quiz twice.

The first time, think about how you were at your best, when you were fit and well and had lots of energy. The second time, think about here and now. In this way you can see what has changed and you can compare the outcome for your prakruti and vikruti.

If one or more Doshas are elevated and at the same time

Ama is present, there is a basis for disease development and it should be dealt with quickly at this point.

The best way to do this in the first instance is to counteract the respective Dosha through our diet and lifestyle (more on this later) and strengthen our digestive fire so that Ama can be metabolised.

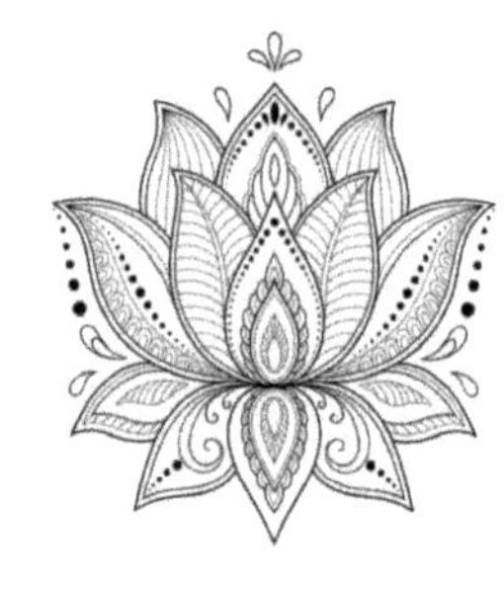

Agni Deepana

Strengthening Your Digestive Fire

As we can see, our overall health rests on the proper functioning of our digestion, and digestion begins with Jathara Agni.

So, the first step in improving our digestion is to strengthen Jathara Agni (Agni Deepana).

To do this, we first need to regulate our appetite. Hunger and proper appetite are the body's way of telling us that the systems are ready to digest. Without hunger, digestion is not going to be at its best.

Practically, this means:

1. Listen to your feelings of hunger. Don't eat when you have no appetite (or at least eat very light food only if you think you need to), but also don't skip a meal when you are hungry.
2. On a daily basis, try to eat at regular times. If your body knows when it can expect food, Jathara Agni will ignite much more easily.

3. Create your routine around your constitution. If you are a Kapha, you might eat one meal a day, plus one or two smaller snacks. As a Vata, you might eat five smaller meals and as a Pitta, you might need three full meals a day. Even if you are cooking for a larger family, it doesn't mean you will have the same portions and the same number of snacks as everyone else.

4. Use digestive spices and herbs (see below) in your cooking to increase Jathara Agni.

5. Chew your food well and eat mindfully, without distraction. Be aware of each taste and enjoy it. This may seem like some old, "chewed-up" advice but if you actually practise it for a while, you will notice a huge difference in your digestive well-being.

6. Eat the biggest meal when your Agni is strong and a lighter meal when it isn't by living and eating according to its biological rhythm. (See Living in Harmony with Nature.)

7. Eat what stimulates your appetite. Of course, if you mostly love cakes and pastries or heavy roasts and pies and bacon sandwiches, then you may have to retrain yourself a little bit first (don't worry, this doesn't take long – soon you'll be craving lentils and greens). But forcing yourself (or your children) to gulp down something you don't like only because you think you should isn't going to stimulate your digestive processes either.

8. Avoid extreme flavours like sugar or very spicy or salty foods. This will also help your taste buds to recover and adjust, so that you will soon be craving

fruit and vegetables instead of crisps and chocolate (yes, this does happen!).

9. Get enough exercise. This increases your metabolism and keeps it functioning properly. Yoga postures are often designed to increase Agni and improve metabolism so that proper detoxification can take place.

10. Eat mainly whole, gently cooked, seasonally available plants and take animal food (meat, eggs and dairy products) as supplementary food, depending on the climate and constitution – some may need more or less of it.

11. Alcohol, sugar, coffee and white flour should really only be taken in small quantities, on holidays or as medicine.

Digestive Herbs and Spices

Kitchen spices have always been used to both enhance the flavour of your food and to aid digestion.

Most of them are warming and increase the digestive fire; some of them are cooling. The following spices are generally good to use for all Doshas but Pitta should use them to a lesser amount, while Kapha can use them quite liberally.

It's important to use good-quality spices. If you want them to have any real medicinal effect, try to buy them whole and either use them as they are or grind them yourself. Spices that are ground up and stored for a long time lose a lot of their properties and are not as flavourful. They also last much longer in their whole, natural form.

Ajwan

Indian celery seed. Very good for Vata and Kapha but – like most spices that strengthen Agni – it may aggravate Pitta if it is used in excess. Heating.

Use it if you experience gas, pain, or nausea but don't use if there is hyperacidity.

Cumin

Cumin is a cooling spice and one of the best to use for all Doshas. It helps all digestive disorders, including gas and bloating. It strengthens the liver and helps the absorption of food and the elimination of toxins. It is one of my favourite spices and I use it often and liberally.

Turmeric

Turmeric is also good for all Doshas, especially Kapha. It's good for digestion, flatulence and works as a tonic for arthritis. It reduces gas and has anti-inflammatory properties. However, for Pitta disorders, it is always best to use turmeric with other spices in a formula, or in a cooling, soothing carrier like coconut milk. If you can, get the fresh root.

Ginger

Dried ginger is more heating than fresh. Fresh should be preferred whenever possible, especially for Pitta disorders. Ginger improves digestion, absorption, and circulation. It's good for nausea, sluggishness, flatulence, migraines, and indigestion. Generally, it is great for all Doshas, particularly Vata and Kapha.

Clove

Good for Vata and Kapha but it can increase Pitta if it is taken in excess. It's good for digestion and helps with sinus/bronchial congestion, colds and coughs, low blood pressure and low energy. It's also an aphrodisiac.

Coriander seeds

Coriander is great for all Doshas but don't take too much if you have a Vata aggravation. It is great for digestion and good for cooling fever and inflammation. It's good to use for hay fever and allergies, rashes, urinary tract infections (it's also a diuretic) and indigestion.

Fennel

Fennel is tridoshic. It's digestive and diuretic, anti-inflammatory and mildly expectorant. It relieves parasites and haemorrhoids and is good for indigestion, flatulence and coughs. It is also easy to grow even in colder climates.

Cinnamon

Cinnamon helps to balance blood sugar and is great for digestion and circulation. Its warming effect particularly helps Vata and Kapha but it can aggravate Pitta if taken in excess. It's great for people with diabetes and sugar cravings and helps with menstrual cramps. It also helps to reduce toxins.

Black pepper

Black pepper is heating and great for digestion. It's good for Vata and Kapha but can increase Pitta if taken in excess. Like cinnamon, it's a great, warming spice for winter. It is energising, increases metabolism, aids weight loss and also helps with coughs, congestion and fever.

Cardamom

Cardamom decreases Vata and Kapha but can increase Pitta if taken in excess. It's good for digestion, coughs, asthma, indigestion, haemorrhoids, and urinary problems. It's also a good tonic for the heart and liver.

Nutmeg

Nutmeg is warming and helps the absorption of nutrients. It's great for anxiety and insomnia and works as an aphrodisiac. It can be quite heating, so be careful if Pitta is already high. If taken too much, it can cause drowsiness.

Salt

Salt is also a great digestive and helps flush out toxins. Use good-quality natural rock salt or minimally processed sea salt instead of highly commercial salt with additives or that has been bleached. Sea salt is more heating than rock salt, though, and too much of it can aggravate Kapha as well as Pitta.

Sugar

Sugar should be used sparingly. Avoid white processed sugar altogether. Instead, on occasion, use jaggery or raw cane sugar which can be great to calm Vata. A little bit of maple syrup is best and Pitta and Kapha should stick to honey as a sweetener if possible.

Ama Pachana – Eliminating Toxins

If you eat just the right amount of food that is easy on your digestion, and manage to keep your Dosha in balance, Ama should be eliminated from your body without any issues. The body knows how to do it; there is usually no need to help it along.

But in our modern lifestyle, it's all too easy to accumulate too much Ama in our system. Maybe we've been eating too much, or too many things at once, or maybe we've been eating foods that are not suited for our constitution or are hard to digest. If Ama has accumulated, there is a lot we can do to support our body's own detoxification processes. First of all, that means we need to stop adding more. All we have to do is take a step back and let the body catch up with its work.

Depending on the severity of the issue, as well as on your constitution, a day, or even a week of fasting can do wonders for your health.

When I say fasting, I don't actually mean fasting.

In most cases, Ayurveda does not recommend a complete, water-only fast. It is usually better to be gentle on the body. A few days of eating very lightly and making use of digestive spices and herbs can be enough to reset your metabolism and immune system if it's done at the right time.

The focus should be on strengthening our Agni and rebalancing our microbiome rather than interfering too much, so that elimination of toxins can happen naturally and easily.

It means eating only very simple food for a while. Food that is very easy to digest while still sustaining our energy and giving us all the important nutrients we need.

Of course, every culture has its own special recipes that are well suited for this purpose. In my childhood, for example, it was chicken soup. In my memory, whenever I was sick, my mother made a big pot of chicken soup, with a whole chicken and big chunks of root vegetables. My grandmother had rusks soaked in tea. In other cultures, there might be porridge, rice soup or dried, soaked bread. This kind of soft food often resembles baby food – simple and mushy and, above all, very easy to digest. The point is to unburden the digestive system as much as possible so that our Agni is used to burn toxins instead.

Kitchari is the Ayurvedic version of such a dish:

Kitchari – Medicine in a Bowl

A typical Ayurvedic detoxification cure consists of eating only kitchari for a few days, taking certain medicinal herbs and performing regular self-massages yourself with warm oil (or having a massage if you have the possibility). Such a cure is gentle and completely harmless – however, due to the increased detoxification processes, it should be avoided during pregnancy or menstruation. If you have a severe eating disorder or malnutrition, it is not necessarily advisable to restrict your diet even more. And for anyone suffering from a serious health disorder it is best to talk to a doctor first.

The Kitchari cleanse can also be done seasonally, twice a year (spring and late summer), as a preventive measure to support the immune system and keep the metabolism balanced.

Over the summer, Pitta increases in the form of acidity and heat in the body, which means that we can become more prone to inflammation, allergies and hyperacidity in late summer and autumn than at any other time of the year. At the beginning of autumn, when the slow cooling and the rising humidity in the air help to release the acid again, we can easily expel it from the body with a gentle Kitchari treatment. If we do nothing, it could, over time, spread through the body and settle in weak spots and eventually lead to more serious problems. If we detoxify right away, we will be much less likely to get infections in the winter and be less prone to allergies.

In contrast, during the cold, wet winter season and the feasting we all do in December, Kapha accumulates in the body. At the end of winter, we often feel weak, tired and heavy from all the Ama that has accumulated – we call this the spring fatigue. The slow warming of spring gently melts the excess Kapha and Ama in the body, making this an ideal time to purify. Spring has always been a time for fasting and detoxing and it is a tradition worth upholding.

There are many variations of this tradition, of course. Depending on our culture, the type of our symptoms and our constitution, we can choose from chicken soup, rice soup, gruel or soaked bread, as long as we limit ourselves to one single recipe for a few days.

Personally, I have always had very good experiences with the traditional Ayurvedic method.

Kitchari consists of mung dhal and basmati rice, and a mix of digestive spices, cooked together to form a savoury porridge or soup (depending on the thickness you prefer). It is mushy, tasty, easy to digest and extremely comforting.

It makes a great light dinner with a small amount of ghee and some fresh herbs, like parsley, chives or coriander. If you wish, you can add some vegetables too.

The Ingredients

Mung dhal

Mung dhal are the tiny hulled, yellow seed of the mung bean. They contain plenty of minerals, vitamins, proteins, and carbohydrates, have anti-inflammatory and gut-soothing properties, and are extremely easy to digest, even for those who otherwise have difficulty digesting pulses.

Basmati rice

Basmati rice is also easy to digest. It may be less nutrient-rich than whole, brown rice but if our aim is the elimination of toxins, digestibility is of more importance. There are also plenty of other types of white (easy to digest) rice but basmati rice, due to its lower glycemic index, is most suitable for all the Doshas.

Ghee

Ghee is purified butter. It contains a lot of butyric acid, a short-chained fatty acid that is also created by the microbes in our gut. Butyric acid is responsible for about 70% of the energy needed by our colonic cells. For thousands of years, ghee was used to heal the gut and improve digestion, and to nourish our bodies inside and out.

Ghee is used a lot in Ayurvedic cooking and healing and it would be difficult to find an appropriate substitute for it.

However, if you would prefer your kitchari to be completely plant-based, you can, of course, leave it out.

It is also often used as a carrier for medicinal herbs and formulas (like triphala). Using ghee with triphala makes it more suitable for Pitta and Vata disorders.

The Recipe

Mix 1 cup mung dhal with 1 cup basmati rice. If you have time, soak it for a while or overnight but it works well without soaking too. Wash it well.

Blend a piece of fresh ginger (and 2 tbsp grated coconut if you like, for Pitta) in a little water. Add 8 cups of water, plus the ginger/coconut mix to a pot, together with the rice and dhal. Cook it on low heat for about an hour, until it is soft and mushy. It will have the consistency of a porridge. If you prefer it more like a soup, simply add more water. Roast 1 tsp cumin seeds and 1 tsp fennel seeds in some ghee, add 1/2 tsp turmeric (and other suitable spices from the list if you wish), and add it to the kitchari. Add some rock salt to taste.

For Vata, add a little extra ghee. For Kapha, don't add anything, but instead, use the spices more liberally.

Use this recipe any time you want to give your digestive system a break.

It makes an ideal dinner. It's light and easy to digest, and it will help you sleep well.

It also makes a good breakfast, if you like savoury tastes to start the day.

You can have it plain or you can add any seasonal vegetables to it to make a full meal.

But if you are using it for a full cleanse, don't add vegetables – keep it plain and simple.

Doing the Full Cleanse at Home

If you are a sturdy Kapha type, you can do this cleanse for up to a week. For a sensitive, dainty Vata type, three days will be enough. Pitta can do about five days.

Choose what feels right for you and don't overwhelm yourself.

In general, it is best not to do this (or any other) cleanse while you are pregnant or menstruating but substituting one or more meals with kitchari to give the digestive system a rest is always safe.

Preparing for the Cleanse

Take two to three days before you begin to gently prepare the body. During this time, avoid or cut down on any stimulants like coffee, alcohol, and cigarettes. Eat plain, simple food that isn't processed, like steamed vegetables, fish or chicken, rice, lentils, etc. Avoid red meat, pork, fried food, and dairy. Do some form of gentle exercise you enjoy. Walk outside in nature.

And, if possible, take up some other supporting measures like self-massage, meditation, or yoga.

You can also start to take a small amount of triphala.

Triphala

Triphala is a very common Ayurvedic formula, consisting of three types of dried, powdered fruit (tri = three, phala = fruit) – Amla, Haritaki, and Bibitaki.

Each of these fruits has a particular affinity with one of the Doshas. It acts as a very mild laxative, a tonic for the liver, and it helps to clear toxins from the body while balancing all three Doshas. It's rejuvenating and very safe to take for pretty much everyone.

One of my teachers used to say: "If in doubt, take some triphala".

Don't, however, be fooled by the words "fruit" and "mild" and "safe". It is very effective but it doesn't have a pleasant taste.

Because of its strong taste, which some people find very difficult to take, it's available as tablets as well as a powder but I strongly advise you to take the powder and experience the taste. You will get used to it. Remember that the effect of anything you ingest starts with its taste inside your mouth. Taking the powder is much more effective than swallowing a tablet. A teacher of mine once said that the stronger you are repulsed by its taste, the more you need it. However, if you are very sensitive then capsules or tablets are certainly a good substitute.

When you buy triphala, it's always best to go to your Ayurvedic practitioner. He or she will know a trusted source of good quality. To order online means to take a risk – there are many brands and not all of them are of the best medicinal quality. Some of them are diluted, some of them are mixed in different quantities, and some of them are grown under questionable circumstances, using pesticides and fertilisers to increase production. Some use inferior ingredients to be able to lower prices or are stored for a long time. There's also a difference if a plant is grown wild and harvested by hand or if it is mass-produced.

If you do want to buy online, just make sure that you

research it well before purchasing and, as a general rule, look for an organic brand and don't buy the cheapest one out there.

You can start by just taking ½–1 tsp of triphala at night, before bed. Vata generally needs a little less; Kapha needs a little more. Dissolve it in about 30 ml of hot water. Stir it well, cool it down a little, and drink it.

Triphala can also be used topically – if you have acne or a rash or a swollen joint, you can make a paste with water and apply it to the area. Leave it for ½ an hour (more or less) and wash it off.

If you have a chronic condition and you are just not sure what is best for you, then let a trained therapist guide you. In most cases, chronic conditions such as arthritis, autoimmune diseases, irritable bowel syndrome, fibromyalgia, etc. respond very well to this type of treatment, and I have seen amazing results in clients and in myself, but if you have any doubts, consult your doctor first.

I remember one of my first clients very well. She came to me with a long list of complaints and an equally long list of medications, almost all of which I didn't know at the time. Her hypothyroidism and rheumatic pain were so severe that she couldn't work and could barely keep her eyes open even during our hour-long conversation. I felt quite overwhelmed and was afraid I didn't have enough experience to be able to do anything for her. However, I recommended a Kitchari cleanse for her, along with Triphala and some other Ayurvedic herbs.

About three months later, she came to me again. Full of enthusiasm, she told me how her pain had disappeared, she was full of energy and, with the help of her doctor, had been able to come off almost all of her medication.

I myself was amazed at how profound the effect of a simple, gentle detoxification cure can be.

Important Aspects

How Many Meals a Day

For 3–6 days, depending on your constitution, eat only kitchari. Eat between one and three meals per day, depending on how hungry you are.

Kapha people might be fine with one meal a day, while Pitta might need more.

Keep the meals regular as far as possible and the portion sizes small.

Triphala

Each night, take your triphala. During the main period, take one to two teaspoons in 30 ml water.

Drink a Lot of Water

During the day, drink as much warm water as possible, preferably with a few slices of fresh ginger or a few drops of lime. In the morning, right after your oral hygiene (use a tongue scraper!), it is especially important to drink plenty of warm water first. A good herbal tea of your choice is also a good idea.

Hygiene

Since toxins are mainly excreted overnight through the breath and skin, a good morning hygiene is especially important during this time.

So the first thing you do every morning, before you eat or drink anything, should be to clean your mouth and tongue thoroughly. Use a tongue scraper to remove the tongue coating that has built up overnight, you can get this online or in most good health food stores and drug stores. Then rinse well with warm water. Gargling with a good oil is especially good for getting rid of bacteria and viruses, because they bind to fat. I like to use sesame oil with a few drops of clove and eucalyptus oil for this. You can also get specifically formulated oils for the mouth.

Then brush your teeth with a mild, natural toothpaste.

You can achieve even more by doing oil pulling for 10-20 minutes (more on this later).

Massage

Daily, if possible (or as often as you can), warm up a small amount of sunflower or coconut oil (for Pitta), or sesame oil (for all Doshas) and do a self-massage on yourself. Start at your head (if you don't want your hair to get oily, leave out the oil here), then massage your feet. Go up your legs, then your arms and abdomen. For an energising massage, go from the extremities to the heart; for a detoxifying massage, go from the middle out along the extremities.

You don't have to be a trained massage therapist to do this; simply use your intuition and decide what feels good.

Yoga and Meditation

Try to do some gentle yoga or meditation practice daily, even just for a few minutes. This will help your body greatly with the mental and physical detoxification.

Castor Oil

On the last day, in the evening, take one tablespoon of castor oil or one teaspoon of senna powder. This will really get things going, so make sure you have quick access to a bathroom!

Castor oil is used quite commonly in Ayurveda. It is a strong purgative and best to use for Vata. It takes a few hours to work, so in most cases it's best to take it before going to bed so that you have a great elimination experience in the morning.

Senna Powder

Senna is great to use for Pitta or Kapha people. It also is a strong purgative and works best overnight.

Your Shopping List

Basmati rice
Mung dhal
Fresh ginger
Turmeric
Coriander
Cumin
Desired herbs and spices to make tea
Dried coconut (optional, for Pitta)

Triphala

Ghee

Castor oil or senna powder

Sesame oil (tridoshic) or sunflower/coconut oil (Pitta)

Tongue scraper

After the Main Cleanse

On the first day after you've taken the castor oil or senna, have a light porridge or rice pudding for breakfast. Later on, add some vegetables to your kitchari.

On the following day, eat as you normally would, but don't go mad! Give your body time and enjoy the new feeling you'll have in your body.

I have come to really appreciate this cleanse as an effective way to reset my digestive and immune system and help to ease off any symptoms that may have been accumulating. I've also seen some quite incredible changes in clients who have done this cleanse to ease their chronic disorders. I believe that it is very safe as long as you don't do it for longer than the recommended period but if you are having some serious health problems or had recent surgery, check with your doctor first.

Kitchari makes a great light lunch or dinner. You can add it to your menu as often as you can. Substituting even just one meal with it will help your digestion already, so try to make it a staple.

I suggest you think of other easy-to-digest dishes like chicken soup or vegetable soup and add those more and more into your routine as well. The more you look after your digestion on an everyday basis, the less you will need long cleansing periods.

It also helps to leave longer periods between meals for digestion until you are really hungry again. In the majority of cases, it is not necessary to buy any over-the-counter medications or remedies at all, if you follow this simple method of detoxification regularly and give your body time to digest. My best advice is to get to know and trust your body, because it will always tell you what it needs.

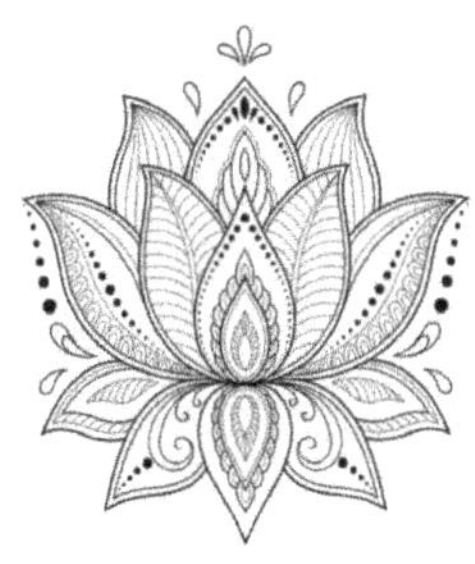

Living in Harmony with Nature

We do not live separately from the world around us, but are in constant, unconscious communication with the world around us. The fluctuations of our physiological and mental functions depend strongly on the influences of our environment. While our nervous system responds to every sensory stimulation, no matter how subtle, our microbiome is also influenced by our surroundings.

The air we breathe, the food we eat, the climate and season we live in, and even the company we keep all affect the balance of our microbiota. The health of the microbiome of the soil in which we grow our food is directly related to the health of the microbiome in our gut. Even the times of day and the influences of the sun, moon and, yes, even the planets affect our minds and bodies.

The philosophical concept of being one with the universe is actually a very real and practical concept – everything really is connected. Just thinking about how many influences come into play at any given moment can be overwhelming. How many people, in how many countries, how many animals and plants have played a role in the production of the dinner on our plate, for example, or in the production of our mobile phones and computers? And how many influences have been affecting each and every decision we ever made? How many events, in a chain reaction of action and consequence, have led to this very moment in our lives and how many other people were involved in it?

We are all made up of the molecules of extinct stars. The same water flows in us that already made up the primal oceans. Any single one of our actions will, at some point, have an impact on the lives of people unknown to us on the other side of the world.

We are all made of the same atomic matrix of charged particles and we experience ourselves and the world around us through the same cosmic consciousness – only from a variety of different perspectives. When we take a walk and admire a plant, an animal or a beautiful colourful sunset, it is as if the same cosmic consciousness is admiring itself in its infinite diversity. We are all indeed one and inseparably connected.

Seasonal Rhythms

The atmospheric pressure, the gravitational pull of the moon, the temperature, the humidity, the strength and direction of the winds – all of it affects us. Everything we experience changes us in subtle ways, causing a reaction in our bodies, either increasing or decreasing our Doshas.

We are literally swimming in all of these vast cosmic energies and it is only logical that we are affected by them more than we may realise.

We all have experienced the different effects of the seasons and the weather on our mood.

Each season has its own Dosha and thus reinforces the same Dosha within us. As soon as it becomes warm and sunny in spring, the energy of fire in the atmosphere increases and Pitta in us also slowly begins to rise. Then in July, when it is hot and the sun shines longer, the Pitta inside of us is also strongest. We may feel this ourselves – many people become more passionate, energetic or even irritable in summer. Our emotions – and also our libido – increase during this time. Especially when we are young, we may experience heightened feelings of love or jealousy, but also more motivation, depending on our Prakruti. And in autumn, when a cold wind blows and the leaves on the trees dry out, Vata increases in the atmosphere. Our body reacts to this is with increased internal movement, transporting accumulated Pitta further through the body, where it can then settle in weakened tissue cells. This can manifest as inflammation, allergies or digestive problems. It is, however, also a very good time to take advantage of the increased mobility of Pitta and eliminate it through a Kitchari cleanse.

This pattern repeats itself throughout the year. One Dosha is enhanced by the atmosphere and weather and then influenced by the next. After Vata has increased in autumn, Kapha can then cause it to stagnate with its properties in winter and so it settles as dryness and stiffness in our bones and joints.

We can prevent this by becoming aware of the influences of the seasons and adjusting our lifestyle accordingly.

And, of course, every country and climate is a little different. Ireland, for example, is generally wetter, colder and windier than most other European countries and has a Kapha and Vata influence almost all year round. People who were born there and have lived there for generations are likely to have more Pitta in their innate constitution. Their skin is fair and freckled and sensitive to the sun, and their digestion is used to a meatier diet because their genes have adapted to living in a colder, darker climate.

Someone, on the other hand, who comes from a hot, dry climate, such as Egypt, will also have developed a corresponding genetic constitution. His body and hair will be drier, darker and curlier and he will filter the sun more through a melanin-rich skin (a typical Vata trait). So when we move from one climate to another, we need to consider our Prakruti and take special care to maintain our balance.

Nature is all around us. We just need to go outside and feel it. Living in harmony with the seasons not only brings us closer to nature – and thus to ourselves – but it also helps our body to better maintain its inner balance.

Of course, this must also be reflected in the food we eat. In most cases, we just have learn to trust nature. When Pitta is at its highest, at the end of summer, we also get an abundance of sweet, Pitta-reducing fruits, vegetables and grains.

In winter, we feed mainly on our preserved foods – pickled fruits, pulses, grains and meats – nourishing, grounding and warming to keep our Vata and Kapha in balance. And at the end of winter, when the first spring greens arrive, we are provided with the ideal plants to help us detoxify and release accumulated Kapha and Ama.

It is easy for us these days to buy a variety of spices and exotic ingredients that are not native to our environment.

This is generally a good thing, as it gives us a much wider choice of food and medicine, especially for those of us who live in colder climates. But I think it's also important that we don't lose sight of our own traditions. Eating what is available to us locally and respecting the traditions of our ancestors by recreating the recipes of our mothers and grandmothers every now and then is as important for our physical health as it is for our spirit. It provides us with connection to our original nature and ancestral roots. And with a little creativity, many recipes can easily be made healthier and more digestible.

Connectedness needs to be felt. The sensory memories of our childhood favourites, the sight of pumpkins in autumn and apples in October, or the smell of fresh wild garlic in the forest in spring can give us a sense of belonging and remind us that nature isn't just all around us but that we are a part of it.

Ritucharia – Seasonal Rituals

At the time of the summer solstice in June, Pitta is at its highest in our atmosphere. What grows and thrives now in our general latitudes are many kinds of green, watery vegetables like squashes or zucchini, salads, berries and potatoes. These are all balancing for Pitta and Kapha, which has been accumulating during late winter and spring, and we should eat them in plenty.

Then, in late summer, after Pitta has been building up in our bodies, there are the particularly sweet, carbohydrate-rich vegetables such as pumpkin, sweet potato and corn. Many grains are also ready for harvesting now. Carbohydrates are cooling for Pitta.

In autumn, Vata increases. Now the fatty nuts are ripe and hunting season begins and we will naturally eat more meat and protein or fat-rich foods. As Pitta is now easily transported out of the body, now is a good time to do a Kitchari cleanse where needed.

In late autumn and winter when it gets cold and icy, Kapha rises and our digestion becomes stronger, so we can take our winter foods like meat, nuts and seeds, dried fruits and grains, and calm down pent-up Vata.

Later, in spring, Pitta slowly rises again and helps to melt the accumulated Kapha of the winter season. Now many supplies are used up, but there are already fresh, detoxifying green plants that we can use for our spring cleanse.

Dinacharya – Daily Rituals

Even every single day goes through different phases, depending on the strength and light of the sun. When the sun is at its highest, Pitta rises in the atmosphere, which of course means that it will also increase in our bodies. It would therefore make sense to eat the biggest meal of the day at midday, when our Agni is naturally stronger due to the increased Pitta. The cycle of the sun continues to determine the cycle of our metabolism.

At sunrise and sunset, and in the early morning hours when everything is cool and calm, we can feel the gentle, cooling Kapha qualities. Now is a good time to meditate or do some other kind of spiritual practice or yoga, or even to express love, either romantically or simply by being with your family.

In the afternoon, the increased Vata in the atmosphere

will enhance our creative energy, which we can use in our activities. To counteract an increase in Vata, it is a good time to rest, if possible, take a relaxation journey or perform some breathing exercises.

Sleeping in the dark and getting up at dawn are natural parts of our biological clock and if we manage to adapt to this rhythm as much as possible, we will soon feel the benefits of it in an increase of energy.

Of course, because of our different working hours, we don't always have the luxury of sticking to these recommended routines. But even if we change just one small thing and introduce a balancing evening routine, which involves switching off all devices an hour before bed, the quality of our sleep will improve significantly.

Taking a relaxing bath, drinking an Ayurvedic warm milk (see recipes), meditating, practising pranayama or even reading an inspiring, relaxing book before bed is far better than watching an exciting thriller on TV or sitting at the computer late into the night.

Even if we are bound to unfavourable working hours and have no way to change it, we can at least do something to mitigate the damage.

Not just the sun, but the moon, too, influences our cycle.

Our cells change their mineral balance with each full and new moon and our hormones are also affected.

Going outside in the morning to greet the sun or to look at the moon and stars at night, even if only for a few moments, is a very simple act, but one that can subtly strengthen our sense of connection with nature.

The Energy of Food

Food, just like our bodies, isn't just its outer form and its energy isn't simply a quantifiable amount of calories. Fresh food is alive and consists of subtle qualities of energy in different forms. These energies are the subtle essences of Kapha, Pitta and Vata – Ojas, Tejas and Prana.

If we want to sustain, or even increase Ojas, Tejas or Prana in us, if we want our vitality and immunity to be strong, then we should be choosing food with those same qualities.

There is obviously a big difference between an organic potato, freshly dug out from the soil and a potato crisp from a factory, or between an apple, ripened in the sun and plucked from the tree, and a carton of concentrated apple juice.

There is also a difference between fresh, seasonal vegetables and canned or frozen ones.

And there is a difference between a mango that has been picked, unripe, and has been lying on a shelf for several weeks, and some freshly harvested, local blackberries.

Try and look at food from the perspective of nature. What kind of energy does it carry?

Is it whole and unaltered? Is it vibrant? Is it sun-ripened? Has it been grown in healthy soil?

Plants also possess cosmic intelligence. They too are a type of consciousness that, in the big universal field, unites with ours.

For those who can't really imagine this, I recommend doing Masaru Emoto's rice experiment once (instructions for this are available on YouTube). I have done it myself many times with my children and can confirm that – if it is done right – it really works every single time.

A small amount of boiled rice is stored in two separate, clean jars. On each of the jars, stick a label on which you write a word – "love" (or another positive word) on one jar and "hate" (or another negative word) on the other. Every day, these words should now be spoken out loud – like you mean it – to the rice in the jar. Children are really good at this! After a few weeks, very clear differences become apparent. The "loved" rice will still be white, perfectly fermented, while the "hated" rice will have turned mouldy and green or brown. Go ahead and try it out, to see the results are really worth the effort!

And since our bodies, like our food, are mostly made up of water (and that's ultimately what this experiment is all about), we can perhaps better imagine the effect of thoughts, words and experiences on us, too.

Our food is also a carrier of different types of energies, which we will absorb every single day.

Of course, this does not mean that we should only eat raw food. Our digestive enzymes cook our food in a certain way anyway. So gentle cooking only prepares our food optimally for digestion. Unless we have a very strong metabolism and a robust constitution or our food is very well "pre-cooked" by the sun in a naturally hot climate, we should in fact eat very little raw food, and if we do, then mainly during Pitta times when digestion is at its strongest. Cooking is like pre-digestion. It takes the strain off our own digestive processes and the absorption of nutrients and elimination of waste can then go much more smoothly.

I have always been interested in nutrition and have experimented a lot with food in my life. Among other experimental phases, I also practised a raw vegan diet for a while, but I found that while I benefited from it at first, I soon felt quite unwell (of course, at the time I wasn't quite aware of my predominantly Kapha constitution either).

I've noticed the same effect in others too – over time, Vata and Kapha simply increase due to the cold nature of the food. It's a bit like throwing wet leaves on a fire. Over time, it just goes out.

How quickly this happens depends on one's constitution, the season and the climate we live in. I think, as with everything in Ayurveda, it's about recognising that our needs are constantly fluctuating. Sticking too strictly to a particular diet, applying rules prescribed by someone else (or even by our own judging mind) rather than by our body, might prevent us from recognising what we really need.

In any case, the food we choose should be fresh, alive, seasonal and of good quality.

Even in winter, when freshly grown vegetables are not available, we can think about the way our food is preserved.

A dried bean or lentil will still germinate if we water it, but a canned bean will not. Its Prana is gone.

In the same way, a pickle from a jar full of sugar and preservatives is no longer alive, while naturally fermented kimchi or sauerkraut is full of beneficial microbes that nourish and strengthen our gut.

A Word about Meat

Ayurveda recognises that humans have been dependent on eating meat for survival for a long time now and that a vegan or vegetarian diet may not be an option, or even suitable, for many.

In the Ashtanga Hrdayam, one of the main texts on Ayurveda, there is a whole chapter dedicated to the medicinal effects of the different types of meat.

Depending on one's constitution, meats might be prescribed for better health.

But it also clearly states that the energetic value of any given type of meat is to be considered. This includes what type of animal it is, where it lived, and how it lived — which makes modern-day decisions a little harder.

Our world is different now.

Most of our meat doesn't come from animals who are frolicking in their natural habitat until they are caught by a hunter but from an ever-expanding meat industry that sees animals as objects rather than living souls.

For this reason, I was a vegan for many years. However, my needs clearly changed with the arrival of my menopause. It still took a long time before I could allow myself to eat meat again. What finally convinced me, morally speaking, was one of my cousins. He is a hunter. On a visit once, I listened to him with fascination, realising how much more he does for nature, animals and the preservation of their local ecosystem than any vegan I had known, no matter how passionate. Yes, I can understand the motivation for veganism very well. But, for me, especially in our northern climates, there are ultimately better, more sustainable systems for living in harmony with nature, animals and one's own health.

Meat in itself is more or less tamasic because of its decaying qualities. If we want to eat meat that really supports our health from an Ayurvedic point of view, we also have to pay attention to where it comes from. Unfortunately, this would eliminate most of what is offered in modern supermarkets.

Whether and how much meat we eat is an entirely individual decision and depends on our prakruti, vikruti, environment and season – all people are different and no one truth fits all.

Genetically, it is the Pitta people who can digest the most meat. Nordic peoples have adapted to their cold, dark climate and developed the typical Pitta traits: fair skin that is sensitive to the sun, the competitive drive needed to survive in difficult circumstances, and strong stomach juices and digestive enzymes to digest animal proteins well. It is still the fair-skinned, Nordic peoples who traditionally eat relatively large amounts of meat and dairy products and can often digest them quite well.

Genetic Kapha people, on the other hand (often people of Asian descent), digest dairy products poorly and can more easily get by with little or no meat.

People of African descent, due to climate, have evolved over generations into Vata types: their skin is darker, hair dry and frizzy, and the need for fat (including animal) to compensate for dryness is relatively high.

So these basic genetic lineages (prakruti) should be taken into account when deciding whether or not to eat meat.

But in addition to this, there is also the very individual prakruti and vikruti, which determines what is needed most at the moment.

During our childhood, we have an increased Kapha Dosha, during our adulthood an increased Pitta Dosha and after menopause an increased Vata Dosha.

In general, it is best if whole, organically grown plants such as vegetables, grains, pulses, seeds, nuts and fruits make up the bulk of the diet. Meat, eggs and dairy products, as well as sugar, salt and spices, are additives that serve more of a medicinal purpose, whenever they are needed. They can be taken to supplement the plant-based diet according to individual needs. How much you take depends, like everything else, on your climate and constitution, though it rarely has to be much. Small amounts of fish, chicken or game meat or the occasional egg are usually sufficient.

However, I always recommend quality over quantity.

Dairy

The issue of dairy is, in our modern times, an even more difficult subject. In the ancient texts, cow's milk is praised as a healing, nourishing and Vata-calming food. But that was in a time, when cows were appreciated and respected like gods for their milk. Milk was equated with love and cows with loving mothers. The milk was consumed fresh and not pasteurised or homogenised and the cows were not treated with hormones and medication. Modern dairy is one of the hardest foods to digest and particularly Ama-causing. If you do like to consume milk, butter and cheese, I recommend you do so in very small amounts, particularly for Kapha people. Vata probably gets away with it most easily. And as with meat, source your produce well. Local farmers' markets may have artisan goat's cheese or raw milk to offer, from animals that are treated with more respect than those living on a larger farm.

Milk was always considered a sattvic food — however, not all milk can nowadays be given that title.

Unfortunately, times have changed in this respect. Therefore, despite the great praise in the Ayurvedic texts, I generally do not consider milk products to be recommendable.

However, there are two exceptions:

Ghee and yoghurt.

Ghee is pure butterfat that has been stripped of all its milky components. Its healing effect on the intestines outweighs the negative effects, in my opinion. It heals the gut lining and activates the production of good microbes and , given that most over-the-counter probiotics are made from dairy anyway, I would prefer to take this ancient natural remedy instead.

However, it is also important to pay attention to the quality of the butter we use in making it.

Yoghurt is fermented milk in which microbiotic cultures have changed the milk components and pre-digested them, so to speak. Here, too, the advantages outweigh the disadvantages in my opinion, but it is best taken diluted, as lassi for example (see recipes).

In general, Ayurveda recommends eating mainly sattvic foods, that is, fresh, whole, living and predominantly plant-based foods – This is how one achieves a sattvic state of mind. Ultimately, a vegetarian diet is more likely to ensure this than a diet rich in meat. But again, achieving a sattvic state is a matter of individual balance, and so individual needs must be taken into account.

To sum it up:

1. Eat mostly whole, seasonal and (as much as possible) organic plants, like vegetables, grains, lentils, beans, fruit, nuts and seeds.
2. Substitute if and as needed with small amounts

of animal foods, sourced for the best quality and energetic state as possible.

3. Eat regular meals with little snacking in between.
4. Cook your food gently, avoiding frying or deep-frying.
5. Add digestive spices.
6. Take a break sometimes and do a kitchari fast in spring and autumn.
7. Eat for your type.

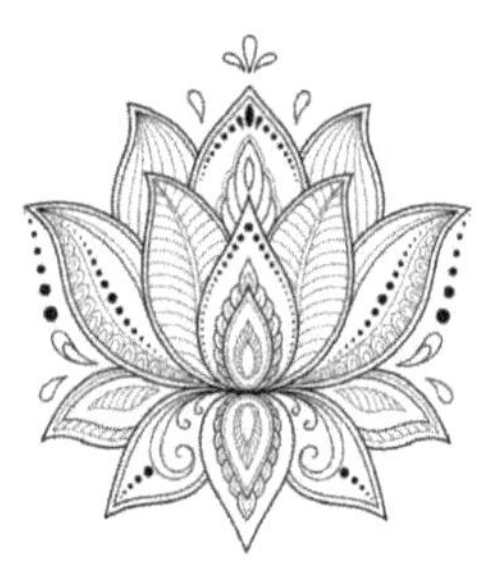

Eating for Your Type

Preenana

Preenana means satisfaction. The more we enjoy our food, the more our body will be open to receive its goodness.

It's of not much use to force yourself to eat something you dislike unless it is some kind of medicine with a purposefully bitter taste.

If you dislike the food you eat, the body will receive subtle messages via your nervous system, and nutrients will not fully be absorbed.

Also, if you feel depressed or agitated with emotions, your digestive system will not be at its best.

You have to feel satisfied from the food you eat for your body to make the most of it. Food is so much more than just functional and necessary. It activates our senses, our feeling of connectedness and it enhances our mood. Eating in the company of loved ones, cooking for your family or friends, or eating food that was made for you by someone who cares about you is priceless. We can't underestimate the value of enjoying our meal.

As always, it's all about balance. Extreme tastes are used as medicine, when we need them. Bitter or astringent herbs, pungent spices, even sugar has a healing, medicinal effect in certain cases. But on a daily basis, we need to keep it balanced.

If we manage to include all six tastes in our daily diet and avoid extremes like sugar or excessive salt or chilli, and if we associate food with a positive experience, then we are much less likely to experience cravings and we will feel more satisfied.

Rasa – The Gateway to Digestion

All our five senses are like gateways to our inner being. Through them, all kinds of information passes through our nervous system into our mind and body. With this realisation, many healing methods have already been developed – colour therapy, aromatherapy, massage therapy, sound therapy and, of course, the Ayurvedic taste therapy.

Rasa (taste) doesn't only exist for our enjoyment, but to give our body important information about the food we are about to digest. As soon as any food touches the tongue, the processes of digestion already begins.

We generally distinguish between six different tastes – sweet, salty, sour, spicy, bitter and astringent.

Apart from extreme tastes such as isolated sugar, salt or flavour enhancers, these indicate what kind of substances are contained in our food: is what we are eating sweet and high in carbohydrates? Or is it salty and contains many minerals? Or is it bitter and cools the digestion? In ancient times, our taste buds were probably much more sensitive than they are today. Moreover, our senses were our only means of scientific analysis and Ayurveda provided us with a very good system to help us keep our Dosha in balance through the conscious use of different tastes.

It is generally recommended to include all six tastes in a meal as much as possible and not to season anything too extremely.

If we eat something that is intensely seasoned with a single flavour, like a packet of crisps or a bar of chocolate, it may seem like a treat at first. But pay attention to how you feel afterwards. Heavy? Nauseous? Thirsty? Tired? Do you have a strong craving for water or for a different taste?

For a food to be truly satisfying, it must have a balanced mix of tastes, nothing too extreme or one-dimensional. And, in general, the more concentrated a taste is, the more medicinal it is and the less of it we should eat.

From an Ayurvedic point of view, sweet taste is present in most foods: rice, pasta, bread, root vegetables, fruit, milk and even meat all have a naturally sweet taste that comes from fat and carbohydrates. The sweet taste is a combination of earth and water molecules found in all macronutrients, which is why it enhances these elements in us, meaning Kapha is increased. This is also important because the Doshas have to constantly balance each other by ingesting and excreting food. But if we consume too much sweet taste, i.e. too much fat and carbohydrates, then at some point we get into an imbalance.

The sweet taste generally dominates our food, but each of the six tastes is important and has a particular influence on the balance of our Doshas.

Madhura – Sweet Taste

* Consists of soil and water
* Mainly carbohydrates, but also fat and proteins
* Increases Kapha
* Has a cooling effect
* Reduces Pitta and Vata
* Is found in many staple foods such as rice, wheat, milk, meat, root vegetables, potatoes, fruit, etc.

Lavana – Salty Taste

* Consists of fire and water
* Mainly minerals, fat and protein
* Increases Kapha and Pitta
* Has a heating effect
* Decreases Vata
* Is found in foods such as fish, seaweed, fermented foods, animal fat and, of course, salt

Amla – Sour/Acidic Taste

* Consists of fire and earth
* Mainly vitamins and enzymes
* Increases Pitta and Kapha
* Decreases Vata
* Found in sour fruits, yoghurt, vinegar, pickles and fermented foods.

Katu – Pungent Taste

* Consists of fire and air
* Mainly found in essential oils and medicinal plant

constituents

* Increases Pitta and Vata
* Decreases Kapha
* Found in onions, garlic and most spices, especially hot ones such as chilli, pepper, mustard and ginger.

Tikta – Bitter Taste

* Consists of air and ether
* Found in most plants, especially green leaves and roots
* Increases Vata
* Decreases Pitta and Kapha
* Found in green leafy vegetables, herbs and spices such as turmeric and also in coffee

Kashaya – Astringent Taste

* Consists of air and earth
* Found in tannin-containing plants
* Increases Vata
* Decreases Pitta and Kapha
* Is found in tea, chickpeas, lentils, pomegranates, apples and pears and other unripe fruits

In our modern days, we rely on our logical mind too often, ignoring our senses, which are a much more direct link to perception and knowledge. Taste can tell us so much more about food than just whether we like it or not. We just have to relearn to understand it.

A balanced meal includes — as much as possible — all six tastes.

Some rice (sweet), some spiced lentils (pungent,

astringent), some green vegetables seasoned with salt and herbs (salty, bitter), and some fermented pickles on the side (sour) are a typical example.

Or, if you prefer it more traditional, think of some lemon-roasted chicken (sour, sweet, salty) with vegetables and well-balanced herbs and spices (pungent and bitter), finished off with a cup of (astringent) tea.

There are many ways to experiment with tastes. If we have been eating a lot of sweets or salty snacks, we may have to train our taste buds again to recognise the more subtle tastes, but once we do, our cravings will disappear, and we will feel much more satisfied with our food.

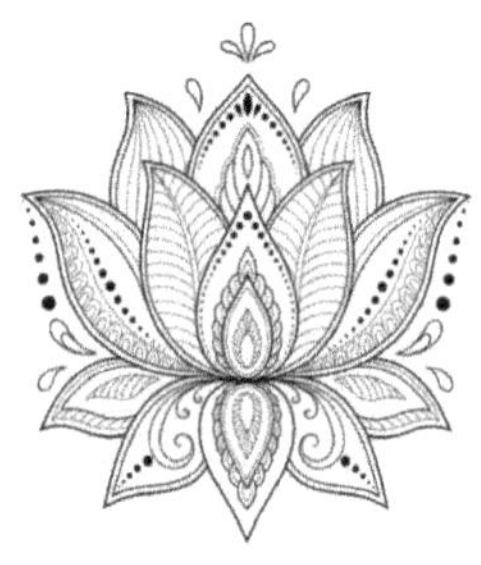

Eating According to Your Dosha

It's always good to remind ourselves again that our bodies are not machines and can't be completely categorised into just one of the three Doshas. But in most cases, one Dosha will be more dominant or aggravated than the others. Recognising these dominant traits will tell us a lot about our type of metabolism. It will give us a good guideline of what types of food are best suited for our constitution.

When we eat for our type, we must take both our Prakruti and our Vikruti into account — our genetic constitution and our current state of health — as well as the seasonal influences around us.

Mostly, and with practice, we will intuitively know what we need. To truly know ourselves means to listen to our body rather than simply following tables. It means opening our inner senses. Even if the mind gets too busy and loud, sometimes, over time, we can learn to listen again to the subtler messages of the body.

The following section is meant as a helpful guide toward a more Dosha balanced diet:

Pitta

Avoid: Fat, spicy, sour, fried food, sugar, cheese, cream, yeast bread.

Enjoy with caution: Dairy products, oils, oily fish, yoghurt, tomatoes, soya, meat, nuts, sourdough bread

Eat as much as you like: Vegetables, especially leafy and root vegetables, sweet potatoes, pumpkin, lentils, chickpeas, beans, white fish, chicken, rice, spelt, millet, barley, fruit, potatoes, ghee, coconut.

Pitta people are naturally hungrier than Vata or Kapha types. So they also need to eat more. Their metabolism is most likely strong and easily converts food into energy. They also need more proteins. Genetic Pitta types, as already mentioned, have developed mainly in northern climates where plant foods have not been so abundant and meat has become a staple. With a healthy Pitta-Prakruti, they can do quite well on a typical northern diet, given that it is of good quality.

However, too much protein, as well as too much coffee, alcohol, fat, fermented or spicy food will eventually increase the already high acidity in the body and aggravate Pitta-type problems such as heartburn, diarrhoea, digestive problems, allergies, autoimmune disorders and other inflammatory diseases.

Pitta people, when out of balance, can also easily become greedy and eat too much due to their large appetite. Obesity is not uncommon in Pitta people who indulge their cravings thoughtlessly. Pitta people do best with regular three meals a day and perhaps a light snack in between when they are hungry. Carbohydrates like white rice or potatoes can be good for soothing an upset stomach and are generally very important for Pitta. I would not necessarily recommend a keto diet to Pitta people in general.

Pitta people overheat easily and therefore need plenty of water, preferably with a dash of rose water or a few slices of cucumber in it. Coconut milk or coconut water is also particularly good because of its cooling effect.

Avoid spicy foods, fried or roasted foods, high-fat foods and red meat – they can increase acidity and make Pitta quite aggravated.

Tomatoes also increase Pitta Dosha, as do overly acidic foods (such as pickles, sour fruits, etc.) and salty foods (such as chips or fries), and should therefore be avoided.

Instead of red meat, white fish and chicken would be preferable; instead of fried foods, choose steaming or sautéing. Instead of chilli, mild, digestive and cooling spices such as fennel, coriander and cumin should be preferred and coffee should be reduced as much as possible. Pitta people may find this particularly difficult – those who cannot do without coffee at all should at least try a milder, less acidic variety and add a pinch of cardamom to it. Sweeten it with a little cane sugar or maple syrup or a dash of plant-based milk, or use ghee or coconut oil to make a blended coffee (see recipes), which eases the stress on the adrenal glands a little.

Ghee and coconut oil are also preferable to use in cooking instead of other cooking oils, as is maple syrup or raw cane sugar (sparingly) instead of white sugar or honey. Those who like to eat bread can choose sourdough bread or Irish soda bread instead of commercial yeast bread. Pitta types can be prone to food allergies or intolerances as they react quickly with inflammation, so wheat and dairy can be a problem for some. It is best to try avoiding these foods for a while and observe if digestion and general well-being improve.

Pitta is not only located in the stomach, but also in the heart and brain, as well as in the eyes and skin.

Pitta types should therefore pay special attention to these organs as they are particularly sensitive to anything affecting them. Visual stimulation, touch and massage, intellectual stimulation and heartfelt passion are easy methods to directly affect a Pitta person.

It would also be a good idea to try to cool down their emotional heat a little more often. Deep relaxation, meditation and cooling yoga practices such as yin yoga, for example, are ideal for Pitta types. They may also enjoy creative forms of stress relief such as dance, art or creative writing, as long as they are not overly competitive.

Walks in nature, especially near water and in the moonlight, have a particularly beneficial effect on Pitta people.

Kapha

Avoid: Fat, sugar, cheese, cream, dairy products, meat

Enjoy with caution: Oils, yoghurt, ghee, coffee, potatoes, bread, game meat, tomatoes, seeds, nuts, coconut, fruit

Eat as much as you like: Vegetables, especially leafy greens, leeks, onions, asparagus, artichokes, broccoli, lentils, white fish, chicken, brown or red rice, spelt, millet, barley, rye, spices.

Kapha people have the slowest metabolism of all the Doshas. This means that they are probably not very hungry most of the time, unless it has been a long time since their last meal. In the morning, they usually need a couple of hours to get their appetite going and, during the day, one proper meal and maybe one or two smaller snacks are often enough for them. Having a slow metabolism is sometimes taken as something negative because it means you gain weight more easily, but you only do that if you eat beyond your capacities and needs. It's actually a very good thing. Kapha people don't have to worry about eating all the time, which saves time and money. It also makes them age more slowly. Kapha people don't dry out as quickly as Vata types, and they don't burn out as easily as Pitta people. And if they take good care of their constitution, they probably won't get sick as often either.

They just have to respect their own appetite and eat only when they are actually hungry, even if this is less often the case as it is with others. However, they are also very social and sensual people who appreciate good taste. They love feeding people, cooking for others and eating together with family or friends. Therefore, it is often not so easy for them to stay within limits.

This is especially true of the high-fat, high-carbohydrate diet of our modern tradition. Kapha people naturally digest carbohydrates well, which is why they love a sweet taste and, if they are out of balance, quickly become addicted to sugar. Diabetes is a typical Kapha disease, which develops by overly burdening the metabolism. It is best to completely avoid isolated sugar, especially in combination with fat. This is easily said, of course, but remember that breaking a sugar addiction is only difficult in the beginning, because as soon as the microbiome and metabolism are balanced again, the craving for it naturally stops.

It is also generally best not to mix fat and carbohydrates in one meal. So, for example, scrambled eggs with peppers or spinach instead of toast in the morning or fish with mixed vegetables and a low GI grain like millet or quinoa instead of potatoes would be great meals for Kapha people.

Large amounts of carbohydrates should be avoided anyway and replaced with more vegetables, especially green ones. Whole grains are better than white flour or white rice (except basmati). Millet is a lovely alternative to rice or pasta. It has plenty of minerals and is easy on the digestion while tasting delicious.

Heavy, fatty foods such as fried meat, chips, etc. should be avoided, as should all sweeteners except honey and dried fruits. Dairy products, especially cheese, butter and cow's milk, are also best omitted and replaced with plant-based milks such as rice milk or almond milk. A small cup of coffee in the morning is actually not so bad for Kapha people, especially if they add a bit of cinnamon to keep blood sugars more stable. Or try a filling blended coffee (see recipes) for breakfast, which will keep the energy up until lunch.

Digestive spices like ginger and black pepper can be used liberally and even a little bit of chilli can be a good stimulant for Agni.

When Kapha is out of balance, it brings a heaviness that expresses itself both physically and mentally. Exercise of any kind is therefore particularly important for Kapha. A short walk after a meal – even just for a few minutes – helps their digestion a lot. Yoga styles such as Ashtanga Vinyasa are well suited for Kapha people. Daily exercise is crucial for their overall well-being.

Kapha is mainly based in the lungs and respiratory tract, mouth and nose and head, so special attention should be paid to these areas.

I know that applying all of these changes can sound difficult at first, but in my experience it is all simply a matter of habit. Once you start eating more according to your type, you will find that it really pays off – you will soon feel so much better in your body that you won't want to eat any other way. Besides, there is so much choice. We live in a time of abundance. For every food we leave out, many new possibilities open up. The trick is to think positively – instead of mourning old habits, look forward to creating new ones. I recommend you buy yourself a good Ayurvedic cookbook and get inspired.

Vata

Avoid: Coffee, alcohol, fasting

Enjoy with caution: Dry snacks, raw vegetables, tomatoes, beans, chickpeas, whole cane sugar, dairy products, cabbage, cold foods, hot spices

Eat as much as you like: Vegetables, especially root vegetables, sweet potatoes, pumpkin, potatoes, lentils, meat, fish, chicken, rice, ghee, nuts, seeds, herbal tea, wheat, barley, sweet fruit.

Sticking to a certain routine and eating full meals regularly may not come naturally to the Vata person, but this is exactly what rebalances you if you are out of whack.

Vata people have a tendency to be dehydrated and deficient. Unlike their Kapha and Pitta friends, Vata people need plenty of rich, fatty and nourishing foods. Good-quality red meat, potatoes and a nice piece of homemade apple pie every now and then are just what this constitution might need. Vata people simply need to be supplied with a lot of nutrients. Their body cells and nervous system need to be well hydrated and nourished to stay in good shape, so it's best not to skimp on good quality fats. Use cold-pressed oils, nuts, avocado, oily fish and ghee, and drink plenty of water, preferably warm. Dehydrating or cold foods such as popcorn, crackers or too much raw vegetables should be avoided and warm, cooked meals with a high water content such as soups and stews should always be preferred.

An extra spoonful of ghee or a drizzle of good oil over your meal helps as well.

Use spices that aid digestion, like fresh ginger and cumin, but avoid too much spiciness as it is even more dehydrating.

Vata is mainly located in the intestines, joints and nervous system, as well as in the ears, which makes them sensitive to sounds and any overstimulation. So routine, enough sleep and relaxation, and regular oil massages are especially important for Vata people.

A good oil massage is not only relaxing but has a profound, regulating effect on the nervous system. By bypassing the digestive system, the nutrients of the oils can reach the nerve cells through the skin and provide strength and balance. The flow of energy (Prana) is also stimulated and promoted by the touch of the hands. A daily self-massage with warm sesame oil can work wonders for an imbalanced Vata Dosha.

Gentle music is also a wonderful means of relaxation for them.

Vata people are sensitive and cannot tolerate a lot of food at once. They therefore need several small meals, which should be kept as regular as possible.

The amount of spices and herbs or medicines they need is also usually less than for Pitta or Kapha people. Unbalanced Vata can also lead to a disturbed or oversensitive sensory processing experience, which also affects digestion. Vata people, with their dominance of air and ether elements, have a harder time than others feeling grounded and staying connected to the body, so it is especially important for them not to stick too rigidly to strict rules, such as following certain diets. These can quickly lead to a negative vicious cycle like addiction or eating disorders. For the same reason, it is especially good for Vata people to preserve cultural and family traditions, at least in part. This grounds them and brings a sense of connection and belonging.

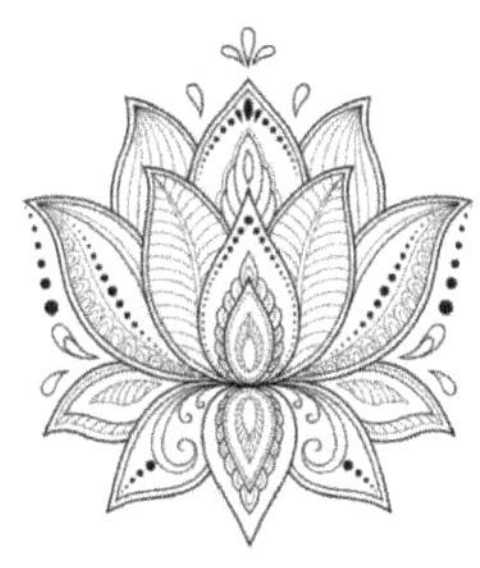

Food Combinations

The simpler the meal, the better it is for our digestion.

Each food needs different types of enzymes and activates different metabolic reactions so it's obvious that combining a lot of different types of foods in the same meal will make it harder on your digestion. It's much more likely that things won't get fully metabolised and end up as Ama in your system if you eat rich and complex meals a lot of the time.

Complex dishes are great for special occasions, but on a daily basis it would be wise to keep it simple.

And, of course, all foods are not equal, and some ingredients work better together than others.

Raw fruit, for example, is best digested by itself and should not be combined with anything else, particularly dairy. So, yoghurt with fruit is – from the perspective of your digestion – not a great idea.

Dairy is particularly hard to digest and doesn't combine well with a lot of other foods like meat and fish. The only dairy that is recommended for most people is ghee, diluted yoghurt (see recipes), or warm, spiced milk (mostly for

Vata). Goat's milk is a little lighter than cow's milk, and easier to digest, but still should not be combined with other foods.

And as already mentioned, it is not so easy nowadays to get good quality, natural dairy that is not full of (artificially altered) hormones, medication and toxins so unless you have a really good source and you are a Vata type, I would suggest doing without it altogether.

Combining a lot of carbohydrates with foods high in fat is also not a great idea, especially for Kapha people. If you eat eggs with toast in the morning, your body will want to use the type of energy that is most easily and quickly available and that means it will digest the carbohydrates from the toast and store the fat from the eggs for later in your fat cells. After a short while, when this burst of energy is metabolised, you may crave carbohydrates again. If you ate the eggs and the fat alone, or with some vegetables instead, your body would have to switch to a fat metabolism, which takes longer and will leave you satisfied for much longer.

As a general rule:

* always eat fruit (except dried fruit) by themselves, especially melons.
* don't mix dairy with fruit, eggs, beans, meat or fish.
* don't mix high-fat foods with high carbohydrates (particularly for Kapha and Pitta).
* use appropriate ingredients and spices to balance out the effect on your Dosha (i.e. add coconut milk, fennel or coriander powder to tomato soup, or pepper, ginger and rock salt to a chickpea stew).

Examples of unfavourable combinations

*   Dairy products with fruit, meat or fish
*   Meat with dairy products or fish
*   Beans with fruit or animal products
*   Fruit with anything else
*   Sugar with fat

Example Meals

Breakfast

Vata – porridge cooked with almond milk and a few chopped dates, topped with a little ghee and a sprinkle of nuts, date syrup and cinnamon OR a baked sweet potato topped with cashew cream or ghee, sesame seeds and a sprinkle of salt and black pepper.

Pitta – rice pudding cooked in coconut milk sprinkled with chopped dates and desiccated coconut and sweetened with maple syrup OR seasonal vegetables (broccoli, spinach, carrot etc.) sautéed in a little ghee or coconut oil, topped with scrambled tofu or chicken/white fish.

Kapha – a cup of blended coffee (see recipes) or, for a similar effect, a cup of coffee with a spoonful of almond butter on the side. This is what I tend to have often in the morning, when I want to exercise or do yoga and don't want to have breakfast but feel in need of energy. It is surprisingly satisfying, and the combination of fat and coffee will slow down the release of caffeine, so the energy lasts longer and is less stressful on the adrenals. Other good Kapha breakfasts are some simple stewed fruit with cinnamon (apples, pear, blueberries, dried fruit ...) or fresh fruit when they are in season.

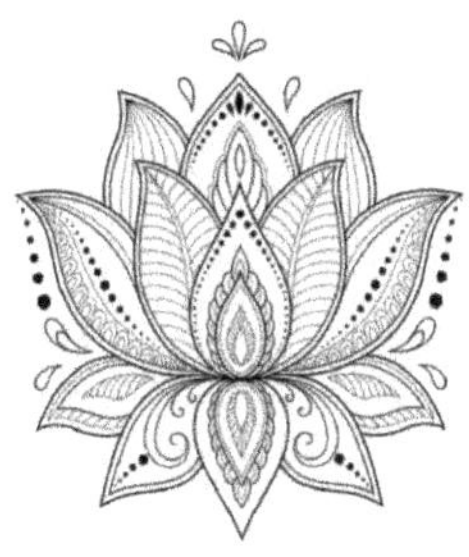

Manas Agni – Mental Digestion

Mental Ama

The same digestive processes that take place in the body also take place on a subtle level in our thoughts and emotions. The "food" we take in through our senses in the form of impressions and experiences must, after all, also be processed, analysed and broken down into its essence, assimilated and then excreted again as active energy, just like our physiological food.

Sometimes, however, our experiences can exceed our digestive capacity, resulting in mental Ama, i.e. stress and trauma.

How we process our experiences and how much of it we can handle depends on our individual constitution. Sometimes a situation that is easy for one person to handle is very difficult for another. Going against our nature is always a basis for discomfort and illness. For a restless, creative Vata person, working in an office as an accountant can be a cause of great suffering, while a Pitta or Kapha person can cope well, even flourish.

A sensitive Vata child may feel more hurt by her parents, judgement or criticism, while a robust Kapha child may not be too bothered by it. In that way, two siblings who seem to have had the same upbringing may have very different experiences. One of them may well suffer from Post Traumatic Stress Disorder while the other may digest the same experience much more easily.

Regardless of our constitution, mental Ama can accumulate either suddenly or slowly, over time. If we overload our minds with impressions through television, news and social media without also eliminating enough, i.e. expressing what we have experienced through our active actions, we put a great strain on our mental digestion. That is why it is so important to express ourselves on all levels, both physically and emotionally, through conversation or creative expression.

Creativity is also the language of the soul and of our subconscious mind. On the soul level, we understand life and ourselves in images, archetypes, sensual experiences and stories. In fact, stories are not only important for children, but for all of us – there is good reason why movies and books are such sought-after commodities.

Storytelling has always been central to human life. All of our ancient fairy tales, myths and legends describe in reality our soul's journey – our transformation from ignorance to enlightenment.

In all of these stories, the hero (the masculine principle, Purusha) embarks on a journey that leads him out of his comfort zone (ego) and into a magical realm (the unconscious mind) in order to free the kingdom (the soul) from some type of threat. To succeed, the hero usually needs a wise mentor as well as allies who can help him defeat the monsters, dragons or demons that stand in the way (our own unconscious conditionings). We all have these demons within us. They are our traumas, our false beliefs and conditionings that are stored deep inside our DNA (the feminine principle, Prakriti). We have to face them, conquer them and recover the treasures they have been guarding – energies that were previously blocked and can now be flowing again.

Only when we can unite our masculine and feminine parts, Purusha and Prakriti, can we become whole. So, in archetypal symbolism, the marriage of prince and princess is not at all anti-feminist, but simply a symbol of the union of mind and body that was previously split off by traumatic experiences.

Every time we read a book or watch a movie, our own archetypes are working along inside.

We need stories because through them we can experience our soul's journey. In some way, we ourselves are basically nothing but living stories.

Our subconscious contains all the emotions and memories we have ever experienced. Many of these are not fully processed and sit as mental Ama in our minds. Every now and then, our subconscious mind, which only ever has our best interest at heart, will present us with one of these unprocessed emotions so that we can remember it and complete its processing. Of course, this leads to the fact that we are often taken by surprise by the negative feelings we experience when we are triggered by something outside of us.

It is then entirely up to us whether we want to accept this challenge and deal with our feelings, or ignore them and blame the circumstances or the people that simply served as triggers.

However, at some point, we will not be able to avoid it. If we really want to be healthy and happy, we have to take care not only of our digestion, not only in a physical sense, but also mentally.

Practising Mindfulness

The external impressions around us never pass us by without leaving a trace. Every impression, no matter how small, that we take in through our senses leaves something in us behind – a kind of seed that at some point takes root and becomes the cause of unconscious, conditioned patterns of behaviour. Whether we live in a green, natural environment or in a big city, whether we watch TV or read books, how our apartment is decorated, and how tidy it is, as well as the kind of conversations we have with our friends – everything leaves unconscious traces. Our senses are truly gateways into our inner world. So we would do well to consciously choose as much as possible which impressions we let in.

This cannot always be controlled, of course, but we can at least ensure in many cases that the "food" we feed our senses is mostly of good, natural quality – going for a walk and taking in the natural sights, sounds and smells, listening to harmonious music or inspiring lectures and stories, reading books that inspire us, etc. will naturally make us feel much more balanced and calm than overstimulating our senses with television, artificial light, loud noises, too much negative news, etc. Obviously, relaxing while watching a horror movie doesn't really work either – our mind is distracted by it, but our senses and nervous system are anything but relaxed in the process.

Simply put, if we keep trying to notice the beauty and goodness everywhere in the world with all our senses, it will have a profound effect on our mental health.

And even the negative feelings that are sure to arise sometimes can be lovingly and mindfully dealt with. If we make it a habit to consciously accept, even welcome and feel all of our emotions in all of their glory, even feelings of fear, jealousy, envy or anger, we will notice how much easier it suddenly becomes to then let go of them.

Dreaming – By Day and By Night

The elimination of mental Ama happens all the time. We speak, we teach, we create, we communicate, we dream and sleep, and we exercise and move. All of this activity cleanses the channel of our mind and increases our mental metabolism. But often the balance between intake and expression is somehow disturbed. Many of us work and study, watch TV and surf the internet daily. But how much time do we take to just be immersed in creativity, play or deeply relax? We need a good balance between sleeping and relaxing (tamas), being productive and active (rajas) and being meditatively absorbed (sattva).

When we sleep and dream, we are processing our mental impressions. But if we don't get enough sleep, our mental Ama accumulates. It is stored in our subconscious mind and affects our behaviour and mental health until it is fully processed at some point. So it is very important to prioritise our sleep.

Depending on the Dosha, we need different amounts of sleep. A healthy Kapha person processes more slowly and naturally needs more sleep than Vata or Pitta people. Women, naturally higher in Kapha, need more sleep than men. When Pitta or Vata Dosha is out of balance, we also need correspondingly more sleep to rebuild the energy lost through stress. A lot of healing happens in our dreams – even if we don't remember them.

Even when we daydream and when we express ourselves in playfully creative ways, we reduce mental Ama. For example, when we write, paint, sing or dance, we express the emotional content of our subconscious mind that cannot be otherwise express.

I am a big fan of journalling. By that I don't mean taking stock of what we do every day or recording our daily routine, but simply writing something off our chest, from deep within, whether it makes sense or not. Putting pen to paper – or fingers to keyboard – and writing for ten to twenty minutes a day, without thinking about it, without pausing, without judging, without deciding what to write, can bring forth surprising treasures from the depths of our minds. Julia Cameron described this method in her book *The Artist's Way* and I have been using it myself for nearly twenty-five years.

The next time you have a problem or need to make a difficult decision, try writing about it in this way for at least ten minutes, without stopping. You may be scribbling meaningless words at first, but if you can engage in the process, you will be amazed at the profound insights about yourself you can gain through this simple method.

Being creative is an essential human need I believe should not be underestimated.

Practising Authenticity

To metabolise mental Ama, as for any other digestive process, we need a strong Agni. Agni is fire, but in the subtle realm of the mind, it is its light that we need, not its heat. It is the light of consciousness that dissolves our dark sides, our hidden fears, unconscious conditioning and behaviour patterns, so that we can free ourselves from an unconscious, mostly reactive existence.

Most psychological problems, from an Ayurvedic perspective, arise from living a life in ignorance of our own truth. Too often we try to fit in with our surroundings, work in a job we don't really like, are stuck in an unhappy relationship and generally ignore the messages of our soul that call for authenticity.

Most of our actions arise from deep unconscious conditioning rather than from our true selves. We keep our head down and we react instead of acting, which makes it difficult to live in a way that would truly make us happy.

To achieve mental health, we need to learn to connect with our true self and live a life of authenticity and freedom. This is, after all, what yoga is all about. *The Yoga Sutras of Patanjali*, the classic text of yoga philosophy, is basically an ancient manual of psychology and mental health. And its greatest goal is to live an authentic life in freedom from unconscious conditioning.

Mental Fasting

Mental fasting means switching off all sensory input for a period of time, preferably on a daily basis.

Deep relaxation, such as Yoga Nidra, and various forms of meditation are methods of mental fasting that allow our unconscious to process pent-up Ama.

A daily yoga practice, if we really do it consciously, is meditation in motion.

There are many traditional methods of seated meditation and most are based on one of two principles: concentration and observation.

In concentration-based meditation, the mind focuses on something like an inner object, a mantra or one's own breath. Through constant practice, we can hold the concentration longer and longer over time until all other thoughts and feelings fade out until eventually only the object of our concentration exists. In this moment, we feel a wonderful bliss that can only be felt whenever we are immersed fully in the present moment.

In the second method, instead of wanting to block out all thoughts and feelings, we allow them, but instead of engaging with them, we distance ourselves from them. We become pure observers, without judging or holding on to any thoughts or feelings. In this way, we gradually become more and more aware that these thoughts and feelings do not come from our true self, but from unconscious conditioning. The more we practise, the more distance we gain and the more equanimous and objective we can then deal with our own problems. Here, too, we will eventually reach a moment of blissful awareness of only the present moment as it is.

No matter which method we choose, I recommend starting very simply, especially if meditation is new to you: one or two minutes a day at first is enough, until it becomes a habit. Then we increase by just one minute every day until we have reached a time that we can sustain well, maybe 20 or 30 minutes. The important thing is that it remains doable for us.

Even an occasional long, leisurely walk through nature, alone and without our mobile phone, can do us a lot of good. A "digital detox" is becoming increasingly important in times of constant digital input. Spending a day or more without technical devices can be challenging, but also enriching.

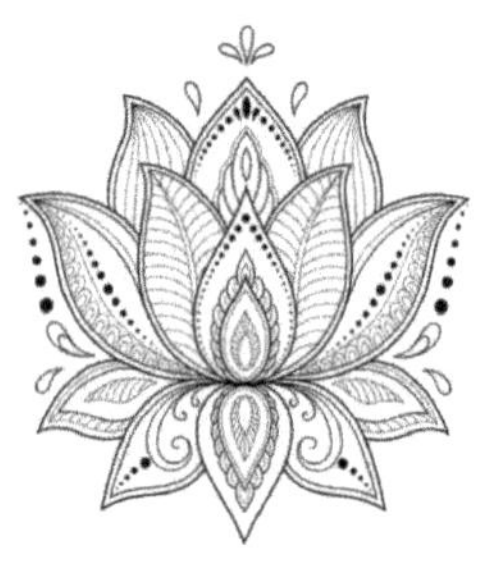

The Pillars of Happiness

Even the ancient wisdom of the Vedas recognises that in order to be truly happy as a human being, four basic needs must be met. These are the four pillars on which humanity is based:

Kama – Love and Sensuality

We are all sensual beings and cannot deny how important pleasant, sensual experiences are for us. The touch of our beloved, the sound of beautiful music, a pleasant, satisfying dinner, the smell of roses in summer or the sight of beautiful surroundings are an important part of our human desires.

Pursuing sensual pleasures is an important and natural part of life. It is not a bad thing, as some religions would have us believe. It only becomes a problem when sensual pleasures are put above everything else or used as a distraction from inner dissatisfaction.

Sensual pleasures calm us and give us a sense of security. They connect us with the world around us and enable us to be present in the moment and to accept and welcome life as it is. Let us try to recall any moment of happiness we have experienced in our lives: when we fell in love, lay in the sun on the beach, listening to beautiful music, etc. All these moments have one thing in common: our environment happened to be so harmonious that we felt we could accept the present moment exactly as it is, with all our senses. We were able to be fully present in our authentic self. Only then can we feel a sense of connection and belonging. Social contacts, friendships and love relationships are also part of this. We are all social beings. We need each other, not just to survive, but to live.

Artha – Prosperity and Health

It is obvious that we all want to be healthy and live safely in a well-built house, eat good-quality food and wear appropriate clothing. It is also obvious that we all want to be able to pay our medical expenses and educate our children.

Our physical needs must be met to a degree that allows us not only to survive, but to achieve full health and vitality.

Without physical health and financial security, it is also difficult to express our full authenticity.

Like Kama, Artha is a basic human need and it is in our nature to want to achieve it. It is important to remember that physical health and financial stability are means that serve a greater good; they are not simply aims in themselves.

Dharma – The Laws of Nature

Nature abides to certain, universal laws that cannot be broken. Water follows a pathway of gravity. The sun sustains life. If we put our hand into fire, we will burn our skin. If we overeat for an extended period of time, we will put on weight.

If we don't live authentically, we will become unhappy.

Just like everything in nature, we too have a task to fulfil in life. Each of us has a special gift, a calling, a role to play in this world to make it a better place. We are all drivers of evolution.

As a mother, I have a duty towards my children and as a daughter, I also have a duty towards my mother. I have a duty to my students and clients and I also have a duty to my friends and neighbours to fulfil. But among all of these duties, the most important one is to myself. It is to fulfil my own calling and become the best, truest version of myself I possibly can be. Our souls are on a journey of evolution – the evolution of the universe. We ARE the universe and we must all follow the universal laws of nature. There is no action without a cause or a consequence. And even the smallest action affects the state of the whole world.

Whether we know it or not, each of us plays a role that goes far beyond our job or family, and that role can only be fulfilled through conscious awakening and authenticity. Only when we ourselves live authentically and follow our heart do we find that calling.

Moksha – Liberation

We can only become truly authentic when we can shed our masks and coloured glasses through which we see the world. By becoming aware of even our deepest, darkest shadows, we can free ourselves from them. This is what liberation – moksha – means: to break free from the unconscious, programmed patterns that hold us back. It is these patterns of behaviour that enslave us, that make us addicted to sensory experiences – to suffering as well as to pleasure – that make us act in ways that do us no good. The true meaning of life, the goal of each of our lives, is to dissolve these shadows in the light of consciousness. If we can transcend our old stories and discard the misconceptions about ourselves, we can recognise ourselves as the divine beings we really are. Moksha – Enlightenment – is the ultimate goal, the goal towards which we are all heading, be it consciously or unconsciously.

The Cycles of Life

Life consists of an infinite number of cycles and rhythms. Like fractals, they arise anew again and again, in the microcosm as well as in the macrocosm of the universe. Our whole life in itself is, in a way, also one long digestive process.

During childhood, we take in physical, spiritual and mental nourishment. We eat, learn and grow. Our water content is high, our muscles and bones grow bigger and our minds are filled with new things to learn. This is the Kapha phase of our lives.

After puberty, we metabolise what we have absorbed. During the Pitta phase of our lives, we work, study, concentrate, are productive and change the world with our activities.

And as we grow older, after menopause, we enter the Vata phase of our lives. This is where we truly need to express our authentic selves. We become wise men and women, the elders, the teachers from whom others can learn. We become storytellers, counsellors, writers, teachers, artists and creators.

These are the natural cycles of our lives and just like the daily and seasonal rhythms, we need to respect them and celebrate them – they are all important to our soul's journey and none is better than the other.

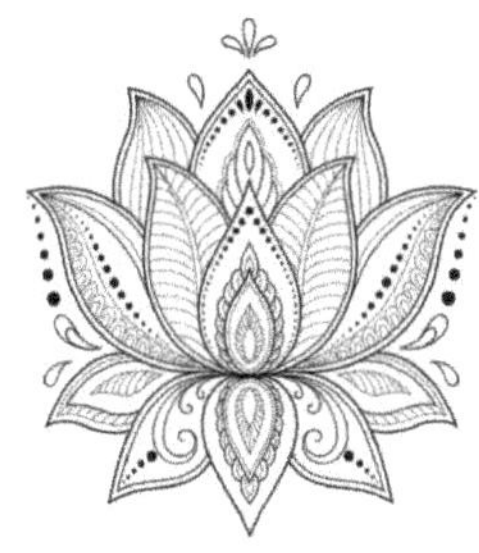

Ayurvedic Home Remedies

These are the recipes that I've been using for myself and my family and that I've been recommending to my clients, with success. They are easy and safe to use at home. However, if you have any health concerns, remember that they are no substitute for a visit to a healthcare professional.

Agni lemonade

Wash or peel a chunk of ginger and blend it together with half a cup of lime juice and half a cup of honey. Add a cup of water and store in a clean jar in the fridge. It keeps for a few days.

Take a shot glass of it before food to kindle your Agni. This is also good for colds.

Cumin honey

Roast some whole cumin seeds in a dry pan, until they release their fragrant aroma. Grind them in a coffee grinder or blender into a powder. Mix this powder with equal amounts of honey and store in an airtight container. Take a teaspoon of it in warm water before or after food.

It also helps coughs.

Pachaka lassi

Mix 2–3 tbsps of good-quality plain yoghurt with 1 glass of water, ½ tsp of cumin and a pinch of dried, or even better, blended, fresh ginger, and some rock salt. Drink after meals.

Spiced chai

Chop or thinly slice about 1 inch of ginger, add to 4 cups of water. Add 5–6 cloves, a few crushed cardamom pods (or ½ tsp ground cardamom), and ½ tsp cinnamon.

Bring to a boil, then add 3 tsp black tea (or the contents of 2–3 teabags). Let it soak for about 10 mins, then strain and add any type of milk you like. Enjoy for breakfast or in the afternoon, or after lunch.

Tulsi tea

Tulsi tea is a great overall drink for all Doshas except for people with very high Pitta. It helps with colds, coughs and headaches.

Ginger tea/Ginger water

Slice about an inch of fresh ginger and simmer it in about 4 cups of water for about 10 minutes. Strain and drink warm or at room temperature.

It makes a great digestive tonic and helps for nausea, headaches and colds.

Coriander water/Coriander tea

Crush 2 tsp coriander seeds and soak in 1 glass of water overnight. Strain and drink first thing in the morning every day.

Helps to soothe Pitta aggravations, inflammation, migraines, digestive issues, heartburn and urinary infections. For Vata and Kaphas it's better drunk warm.

You can also take ½–1 tsp freshly ground coriander powder in ½ cup hot water for acute needs (i.e. heartburn).

Ayurvedic milk

A nice evening ritual is to drink a cup of spiced, warm milk before bed. I personally like oat milk, pea milk or almond milk best. Warm the milk with about a teaspoon of the following herbs and sweeten to taste:

* Cardamom and rose water (for Pitta)
* Cinnamon and cardamom (for Vata)
* Turmeric, ginger and pepper (for colds and increased Kapha)
* Ashwagandha and nutmeg (for sleep disorders)

Rose water/Rose petals

Rose petals are cooling and great for all Doshas, especially Pitta. They work as a mild anti-depressant, aphrodisiac, and sedative. Good for frequent infections, bladder and kidney infections, and urinary disorders.

Use the petals as tea or add rose water to warm milk or rice pudding.

Rose-water flavoured water makes a great, cooling and refreshing drink.

Aloe vera

Aloe vera is also cooling and good for Pitta and inflammation. A mild laxative and rejuvenating tonic, it is particularly good to use for women during menopause and for weight loss. Too much of it can be toxic, so be careful with the dosage. Follow instructions on your bottle, as brands can differ in concentration.

Sesame seeds

Take 2 tbsp of sesame seeds (black, if you can get them) every day for any type of bone tissue problem like osteoporosis or weak teeth, nails or hair. Sesame seeds are heating, so do take care if you have Pitta imbalances. Sesame oil is also the best oil for Ayurvedic massage therapy.

Nutmeg

Nutmeg is an amazing remedy. ¼ tsp of the freshly ground nut in warm (plant) milk at night, sweetened if you like. It helps insomnia and anxiety and acts as an aphrodisiac, especially for men. Just be careful of Pitta conditions as it is heating. Also, don't take more than ½ tsp as it can make you drowsy.

Liquorice

Liquorice is very cooling and great for Pitta conditions like acidity, ulcers, menopausal symptoms, liver problems and inflammatory pain. It also reduces Vata and is good for the nervous system. It can increase Kapha, though.

½ tsp in (plant) milk or water.

Triphala

I've mentioned it before. Triphala is a mix of three different types of dried, powered fruit: haritaki, bibitaki and amla. In my experience, it is one of the best remedies and everyone should have it in their home apothecary. It is safe to use for all Doshas, has a balancing effect on Vata, Pitta and Kapha, and acts as a mild laxative and detoxifier. It is my go-to remedy and first call for many conditions.

Ashwagandha

Like Triphala, Ashwagandha is also a very popular home remedy. It has an aphrodisiac effect (especially for men) and helps with stress. It can be taken in the morning to get more energy or in the evening to sleep better. But caution is advised with very high Vata. Half a teaspoon in hot water or in warm milk in the evening is sufficient.

Shatavari

Shatavari also has an aphrodisiac effect, especially on women. It calms Pitta and can have a hormone-balancing and rejuvenating effect that is very helpful during menopause, but should be avoided if there is an oestrogen intolerance. It also mixes well with ashwagandha. Half a teaspoon in water or in warm milk in the evening.

Ayurvedic Recipes

All the following recipes are very easy to digest and can be used for all Doshas. They are common in Ayurvedic cooking and help to keep a good digestion, metabolism, and Doshic balance.

Use them as often as you like in your everyday cooking.

Mung dhal

Wash 1 cup of mung dhal and boil in 6 cups of water until it is soft and mushy. Use a whisk to smooth it out. In a pan, melt 1 tbsp ghee or oil, and roast 1 tsp each of whole cumin, ajwan, and fennel seed in it, then add some coriander powder and –1/2–1 tsp turmeric. Add the mixture to the dhal, then add rock salt to taste.

If you wish, you can also add some vegetables to this. Spinach or other greens work well.

Vegetable subji

Melt 1 tbsp ghee and roast whole spices like cumin, ajwan, mustard or fennel. Then add powdered spices, like coriander, cinnamon, pepper, ginger or turmeric. Add fresh, chopped vegetables of the season and a little water or coconut milk (for Pitta). Season with rock salt and cook until tender.

Kitchari (see recipes).

As an everyday dish, add whatever seasonal vegetables you like. If you are doing a cleanse, keep it plain.

Porridge

In Ireland, where I lived for 24 years, porridge is a standard breakfast that many children grow up with. I love it myself. It doesn't have to be made with oats either, and it doesn't always have to be sweet. My Romanian grandmother often made "Mamaliga", a type of porridge made from Maize. I still love it, especially topped with some ghee and spinach. Maize is excellent for Kapha people, but spelt semolina, millet, oats, quinoa or almost any other grain can also be made into a lovely, comforting porridge. If you like it sweet, add sultanas, dates or other dried fruits and a little maple syrup, date syrup or honey. Spices such as cinnamon, ginger or cardamom and a little ghee or coconut milk are also great to add flavour. The grains can be cooked either in water or milk, depending on your Dosha and taste.

Rice pudding

Cook ½ cup of basmati rice in a can of coconut milk. Add another cup of water, cardamom, and cinnamon. Cook it for about 30 mins, until it is soft and mushy. For Pitta, add some rose water if you have it. For sweetness, add some chopped dates or any good-quality sweetener of your choice.

Stewed fruit

Chop one or more seasonal fruit into chunks (apples, pears, blueberries, etc.). Add dried fruit such as dates, raisins, or figs (to taste) for more sweetness. Add some cinnamon and/or cardamom and cover with a little water. Simmer until soft.

Chapatis

If you are avoiding yeast, you can make a delicious, yeast-free bread very easily within minutes.

Use either chapati flour from an Asian market or mix 1 part white flour and 1 part wholemeal. Spelt works very well too and is better suited for Kapha and Pitta than wheat. You can add a few ajwan seeds for better digestion and flavour. Mix with water and knead until the dough feels dry and elastic. Shape into a ball. Roll out thinly, using more flour to keep the dough from sticking. Cook on a hot, flat, dry pan, just a few minutes on each side, until it begins to puff up. If you like, you can brush some ghee on each side when it's done.

Rice soup

Cook 1 part rice with 8–10 parts water for at least one hour to make a thick soup. Leftover cooked rice works really well for this dish. Season with salt, ginger, and other optional spices. Add green vegetables and/or top with cooked fish, chicken or egg for a light and easy-to-digest meal.

Blended coffee

A cup or two of coffee is alright for Kapha people if there are no other issues.

For Pitta/Vata disorders, try to reduce or avoid. Because many of us find it very difficult to do without it, here is a way to reduce its aggravating effect.

If you are someone who doesn't like eating breakfast but needs some energy, try this recipe:

To a cup of black coffee, add 1 tbsp of coconut oil, ghee or almond butter and blend very well until it is completely emulsified into a creamy, delicious coffee. You can also add cinnamon or cardamom to the blend.

The fat in the coffee will give you a lot of energy and it will help release the caffeine more slowly. It also will keep hunger away and makes a great drinkable breakfast for Kapha that will keep away the sugar cravings.

Ghee

Use good-quality, unsalted butter. A slow cooker works particularly well. If you don't have one, try a heavy pot that distributes the heat evenly.

Put the butter in the pot and set it on the lowest heat possible. When all the butter is completely melted, you can see the separation of pure, translucent fat and a white, milky substance at the bottom.

Use clean empty jars and slowly pour the fat into the jars without getting to the milky bit. You may have a little bit of waste with this method but I find it is by far the easiest and gentlest way to make ghee.

And the leftovers aren't wasted if you have a dog.

Date milk

Blend a glass of almond milk or coconut milk with 1–5 dates. Medjool dates are much sweeter than other kinds, so one or two are probably enough. You can also add some cardamom. It makes a great breakfast drink or afternoon energiser, especially for Vata and Pitta.

Fig shake

Soak and blend 3–4 figs with water, a spoonful of almond butter (more for Vata, less for Kapha) and some cinnamon. This makes a great breakfast drink for all Doshas.

Herbal stew

Use seasonal vegetables and add either chicken, fish or lentils. Blend a chunk of fresh ginger and a piece of fresh turmeric with water and add it to the vegetables. Season with rock salt, black pepper and fennel, and add some fresh herbs like parsley, chives or coriander. This makes a great tridoshic stew for autumn and winter.

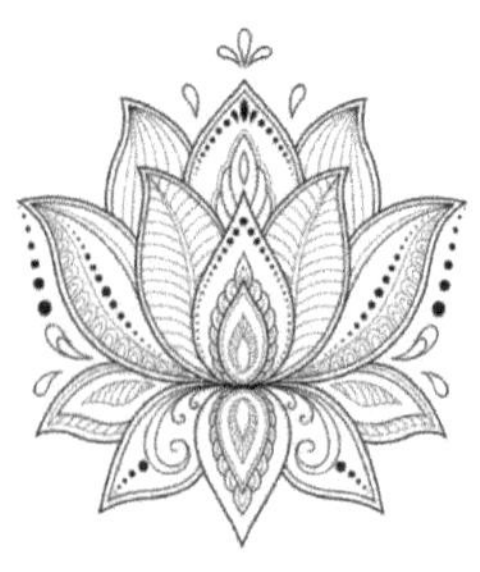

Other Supporting Practices

Exercise

All forms of exercise increase our circulation and keep our Prana flowing. This is important to keep Srotamsi clear and unobstructed.

The more we move, the more our metabolism speeds up. Our blood flows quicker, our synapses fire better, our accumulated Ama is transported out of the body more efficiently and Prana can flow more freely again.

If we move too much, however, we may cross the fine line into creating too much stress on our body, which has the opposite effect – Vata is increased, our nervous system over-stimulated and our stress responses activated too much. It's important to get the balance right. But only you will know what the right amount is. If you are enjoying what you do, and if you are feeling balanced and good afterward, then it is probably good for you – as long as you don't get stressed out when you skip it for a day.

But what's right for one person is not necessarily right for the other.

It is always important to look at both Prakruti and Vikruti.

Our Prakruti tells us about our natural tendencies.

A person with Vata Prakruti may naturally want to move more, with bursts of energy, but tires or gets bored more quickly. They might be drawn to running, dancing or other forms of exercise that require quick responses. But a Vata Vikruti person has to watch out – they will need more strengthening and grounding exercises.

A Pitta Prakruti person loves competition and achievement and needs a challenge. But a Pitta Vikruti person will need to learn how to take things easy and be more playful.

A Kapha Prakruti person will be more drawn to strength-based workouts but a Kapha Vikruti will need to introduce more movement and cardiovascular exercise.

Whatever we do, it's vital that we start where we are at, that we recognise our nature and choose what gives us joy. But we must also recognise our imbalances and move towards our opposite where necessary.

Even if we have never exercised before and have to get used to moving our bodies, we can start slowly, step by step. A ten-minute walk after lunch that slowly evolves into a longer hike is much better than trying to do it all and then feeling overwhelmed.

Walking in nature is a practice by itself and should be done by everyone, regardless of constitution. To breathe in the fresh air, inhale nature's microbiome and soothe the senses by the gentle sights can be more therapeutic than any expensive treatment.

Yoga

Nowadays, yoga is mostly associated with a method of stretching and breathing, focused on the physical body. But in reality, it is so much more.

The Yoga Sutras of Patanjali, the classical text on yoga, is actually a manual on mental health. It is a description of the kind of bliss, well-being and potentiality the human mind is capable of and how we can achieve it. Asana – the physical postures – are only one small (but important) part of it.

Yoga is based on Ayurvedic principles, and a good practice is designed to address issues of Dosha imbalances, to strengthen Dhatus and Agni, and eliminate Ama. It also adjusts the flow of Prana, Udana, Samana, Vyana and Apana Vata and enhances Prana in particular, significant energy points (Marma) of the body. It also works on the endocrine system and organs. This is what is meant by "Yoga Cikitsa" – yoga therapy – in the traditional sense.

The dynamic effort and concentration of the practice (Pitta) should be in balance with its strength and stability (Kapha) and with its movement, breath and spaciousness in the body (Vata). An even inhale and exhale balances our nervous system and a focused mind brings heightened awareness. A daily yoga practice is like spending quality time with our child, or a lover. We get to know our body on the deep level of its cosmic intelligence, where there is no egomind, only the striving towards balance and wholeness.

Practising the balance between flexibility and strength, inhale and exhale, stillness and movement on a physical level will also, in time, calm and balance the fluctuations of our mind.

The traditional first series of Ashtanga yoga is based on Ayurvedic principles and has a balancing effect on all doshas if it is individually adapted and not simply rigidly followed.

And yoga naturally includes focusing on the breath. Pranayama – specific breathing exercises to balance and strengthen Prana – is a very effective way to balance the whole nervous system. It is designed specifically to balance Vata and, by extension, all Doshas.

It's best to ask your yoga teacher about this.

Tongue Scraping and Oil Pulling

A large part of what we eliminate from our body is exhaled as carbon dioxide and in this process, the toxins from our body accumulate on our tongue. You can see it as a thin, white coating that is probably particularly strong in the morning. This coating is normal and a sign that Ama is being eliminated. If there is a lot of it, or if it is of a peculiar colour, we know that there is a lot of Ama in the body. Either way, we want to get rid of it before we eat or drink anything first thing in the morning.

Use a tongue scraper (you can buy one in most health food stores or order online) to gently scrape it off and brush your teeth with a natural toothpaste. When your mouth is clean, drink a glass of fresh water – room temperature or warm – before you have anything else to eat or drink.

In this way, you are supporting the elimination of Ama from the mouth and are assuring proper hydration, without swallowing toxins back into the body.

In the evening, after rinsing your mouth, take about 1 tablespoon of sesame oil and swish it around your mouth vigorously for a few minutes – start with 5 or 10 minutes and work your way up to 20.

"Pull" the oil in between the gaps of your teeth and make sure it emulsifies well with your saliva. When you spit it out, it should have a thick, white consistency. Not only will you pull out a lot of harmful microbes which cling to the fat, but unlike harsh mouthwashes, you will be creating a good environment for beneficial microbiota in your mouth.

Gently brush your teeth afterwards.

Neti and Nasya

The nasal passages are our first line of defence to ward off harmful microbes we breathe in through the air. It is therefore important to keep the nasal membranes and sinuses healthy, nourished and free from excessive mucus.

A Neti pot is a little pot with a snout, designed to rinse your nose and sinuses. You can buy it in pharmacies, health food stores, and online. The pot is filled with warm salt water, which is then poured into one nostril until it flows out the other. This practice helps to keep mucus and bacterial infections at bay.

To soothe and nourish the mucus membranes and nervous system, take a few drops of sesame oil on the tip of your finger or a cotton bud and massage it into the inner membranes of your nostrils (Nasya). These practices will help you stay free from infections and headaches.

Massage

Oil nourishes the nervous system membranes with its fatty acids. It penetrates through the skin, bypassing the digestive system, calms and strengthens the dhatus, and influences the circulatory system and the endocrine system in a positive way. We can feel its benefits almost immediately.

Touch softens and rehydrates connective tissue and can help to relieve tension and trauma from the body. It rejuvenates the whole system.

Massage, in my opinion, cannot be overrated. In many cultures, it used to be traditional to massage children or loved ones regularly – no special training was necessary. Personally, I loved to massage my own children when they were young, and I believe it had a very positive effect on their overall well-being.

I've also had some extremely good results using daily oil massage on children with neurological disorders like FASD.

Nowadays, massage treatments have been pushed into the realm of luxury and indulgence. Once or twice a year, we might treat ourselves to a spa treatment, but otherwise we don't even think about it, unless we are in pain.

Of course, a professional massage is ideal. An Ayurvedic massage therapist will know the best techniques to help the oils unfold their therapeutic effect. He or she will also analyse your constitution and disorder and match their techniques to your personal needs.

However, on a regular, day-to-day basis, you can do so much by yourself. A ritual of self-massage a few times a week will do absolute wonders to keep your Vata in check and balance out your constitution.

To do this, get yourself some good-quality oil – sesame oil is usually recommended for all Doshas (try to find purified, cosmetic grade oil to avoid smelling like food) – and massage it into your skin. Begin at your feet and rub your ankles in circular motions. Use long strokes on your calves and thighs and circular movements on your joints.

Do the same on your hands and arms.

Massage your scalp with oil too. This is not only great for growing healthy hair but also for the circulation and nourishment of your brain.

Massage your abdomen in gentle circular movements, in a clockwise direction.

Give your breasts some attention too, and finish with your face and particularly your jaws.

Let the oil soak in for at least 30 mins (or more, if you have time) and then shower it off.

If you are short for time, do at least your feet, head, and abdomen.

For Vata, use a particularly liberal amount of oil. For Kapha, use only a little, or try some dry brushing.

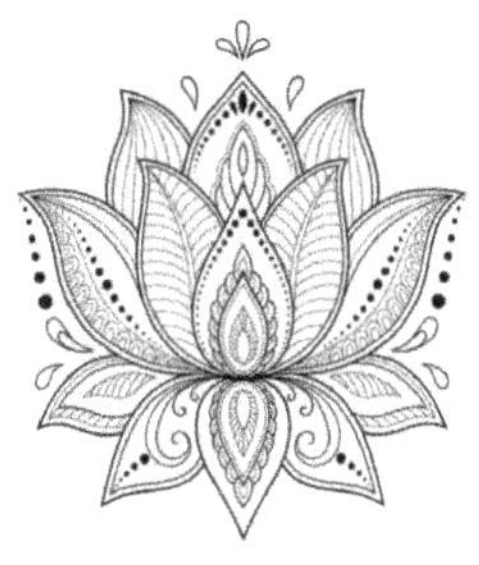

Radical Self Love

One last piece of advice: whatever you want to change in your life, let it be a change that happens out of love.

Our subconscious stores every memory we have ever experienced. Many of them are unprocessed emotions and beliefs that guide our actions – but not always in the direction we want.

As a result, even though we know what we want, we often do the exact opposite.

Of course, there are many ways to free ourselves from such unconscious conditioning, like yoga, meditation or more conventional Psychotherapy.

However, there is one very basic attitude without which real transformation is not possible, and which is actually quite easy to learn, and that is radical self-love.

Of course, I don't mean love for one's own ego, but love for the true, authentic self, which is expressed through the body.

I call it radical, because acting in a way that respects our own body's needs and listening deeply to it's messages, often interferes with the expectations of friends, family and society as a whole. To prioritise loving one's Self requires courage. It means not caring about other peoples opinions anymore and risking dislike from people around us. But when we truly act out of love, we will attract the exact people that will love us for who we really are and the whole world will be a better place for it. As already mentioned, love is the fundamental motivation of all life and is therefore part of our nature.

Love and deep connection are really the same thing.

The more we get to know ourselves, the more we will automatically love ourselves.

And the stronger this connection with the self becomes, the stronger will our capacity for self-care, for loving others, and for experiencing happiness and contentment be.

Only through the practice of radical self-love will our diet and lifestyle improve quite naturally, because then we will want to do something good for ourselves every day all by ourselves.

So the best place to start is by spending quality time with ourselves.

Nurture that feeling of love for yourself and let it grow, because you are an incredible cosmic being, an intelligent, self-healing organism, a microcosm of the entire universe. You are made up of the molecules of suns and stars – you are literally a reincarnation of the heavenly bodies. You are made of stardust and the waters of primal oceans, of energy, light and sound in search of harmony and wholeness.

Your driving force is love, which is reflected in every single atom of your body.

Isn't it time to recognise this and love yourself just as you are, in all of your divine glory?

And when things aren't going so well sometimes, try to remember that life is about the evolution of our soul, and such evolution only happens when there are also stresses, burdens and obstacles. We may not want these obstacles because they are unpleasant or frightening, but in the long run even the worst experiences offer us the opportunity to grow and become wiser and resolve our old karmic seeds that we no longer need.

Life is a journey of discovery. I hope that through Ayurveda you can discover the amazing beauty and intelligence of your body – the expression of your soul – and learn to love yourself exactly as you are.

You can find out more about me on:
www.sandrahayes.eu

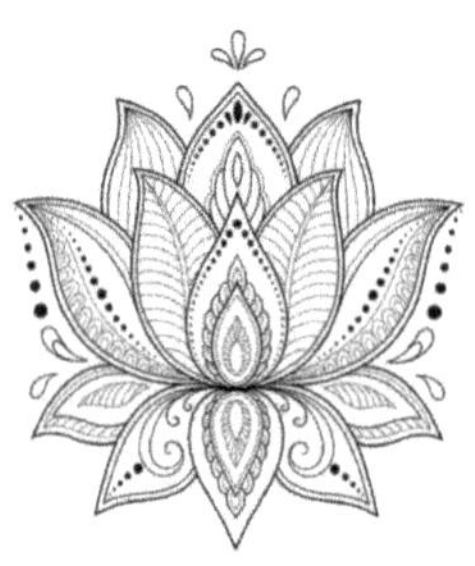

Sources

Online

Satmya	www.satmya.ie
Ayurveda Institute UK	www.ayurvedainstitute.co.uk
The Ayurvedic Institute	www.ayurveda.com
Ayurveda Ireland	www.ayurveda.ie
Zach Bush MD	www.zachbushmd.com
National Library of Medicine	https://www.ncbi.nlm.nih.gov

Books

Vasant Lad *Textbook of Ayurveda Vol. 1, 2 & 3*
The Complete Book of Ayurvedic Home Remedies
Ayurvedic Cooking for Self-Healing
Amadea Morningstar *The Ayurvedic Cookbook*
David Frawley *The Yoga of Herbs*
Ayurveda and the Mind
Chowkhambra Krishnadas Ayurveda Academy *Astanga Hrdayam Vol 1, 2 & 3*

www.ingramcontent.com/pod-product-compliance
Lightning Source LLC
Chambersburg PA
CBHW060749240726

48664CB00009BA/1669